CHAIR YOGA FOR WEIGHT LOSS

CLAUDIA LYNNE

RMC PUBLISHERS

CONTENTS

INTRODUCTION

Are you looking for a gentle, accessible way to improve your health, reduce stress, and increase flexibility? The modern world can be challenging to your overall health and fitness. Most people are pushed into a sedentary lifestyle and spend long hours sitting at a desk. Others may face challenges like injuries or health complications, yet more may feel that traditional yoga, with its deep stretches and complicated poses, is unattainable.

There is, however, a solution that can help you achieve your wellness goals without the need for expensive exercise equipment or advanced yoga skills—*Chair Yoga for Weight Loss*.

Chair yoga is a modified form of yoga that incorporates gentle movements, stretches, and breathing exercises while using a chair for support. This innovative approach makes yoga accessible to people of all ages, fitness levels, and abilities. Whether you're new to yoga, have limited mobility, or simply don't have the time or space for a full yoga practice, chair yoga offers a convenient and effective way to experience the many benefits of yoga.

If you've struggled to find a weight-loss exercise routine that fits your lifestyle and addresses your specific needs, chair yoga is the perfect solution. Practicing chair yoga regularly can counteract the adverse effects of prolonged sitting, such as muscle stiffness, poor circulation, and weight gain. Chair yoga can help you build strength, improve flexibility, and reduce stress and tension in both your body and mind.

One of the most significant advantages of chair yoga is its adaptability. You can practice it virtually anywhere, whether at home, in the office, or while traveling. All you need is a sturdy chair and a willingness to dedicate a few minutes each day to your well-being. With chair yoga, you can easily integrate mindful movement and relaxation techniques into your daily routine, no matter how busy your schedule is.

When reading *Chair Yoga for Weight Loss*, you'll discover the transformative potential of this practice. You'll learn how to perform a variety of chair yoga poses, breathing exercises, and relaxation techniques that can help you achieve your health and wellness goals. Whatever your goals are, losing weight, reducing stress, improving your posture, or simply feeling more energized and balanced, chair yoga offers a gentle, accessible path to success.

As you begin this 28-day challenge, you will learn:

- What chair yoga is and why it is so effective for weight loss.
- How to start with your chair yoga practice, including choosing the right chair and creating a space to work out.
- Step-by-step instructions and accurate illustrations will guide you through each of your poses.
- A 28-day workout program that gradually increases in difficulty as your body adapts and strengthens.
- Guidance on sustaining your chair yoga practice beyond your first 28 days.

The beauty of chair yoga is that it meets you exactly where you are in your fitness journey. It's not about perfection or achieving advanced poses. Instead, in choosing chair yoga for weight loss, you connect with your body, mind, and breath in a nurturing and supportive way. With each practice, you'll build strength, confidence, and a deeper sense of well-being as you begin to lose weight.

So, let's get ready to experience the many benefits of chair yoga.

CHAPTER 1
UNDERSTANDING CHAIR YOGA

*C*hair yoga is a form of yoga that uses a chair as a prop to help you move through modified poses. The simplicity of modifying traditional yoga practices can be deceptive, especially when it comes to chair yoga practices. Chair yoga is a powerful exercise that benefits both body and mind without putting too much strain on your muscles and skeletal system.

However, using a chair to complete yoga poses isn't necessarily a less effective version of traditional yoga. Instead, this innovative approach has been designed to make yoga more accessible and manageable for people with limited mobility or physical limitations or those who prefer chair yoga to traditional yoga —while providing the same benefits of strength, flexibility, and balance.

The History and Origins of Chair Yoga

This innovative approach to yoga emerged in the mid-20th century as yoga teachers sought ways to make the practice more attainable to people of all ages and abilities. The concept of using props in yoga wasn't new, and renowned yoga master B.K.S. Iyengar popularized using blocks, straps, and other aids to help practitioners achieve proper alignment and deepen their practice. Chair yoga took this idea further, transforming an everyday object into a valuable yoga prop.

One of the pioneers of chair yoga was Lakshmi Voelker-Binder, who developed her "Get Fit Where You Sit" program in the 1980s. Inspired by a student with arthritis who couldn't participate in traditional classes, Voelker-Binder created a series of yoga poses that could be done while seated. This groundbreaking approach opened the door for countless individuals who had previously felt excluded from yoga practice.

Since its inception, chair yoga has become popular and evolved to include various styles and approaches. Today, you can find chair yoga classes in senior centers, offices, hospitals, and even airports!

The Benefits of Chair Yoga Over Traditional Yoga for Beginners

Chair yoga offers a wide range of physical and mental benefits that help to improve both the body and mind. Let's break down these benefits.

- **Flexibility and mobility:** One of the primary benefits of chair yoga is improved flexibility and mobility. One study showed that a 12-week chair yoga program significantly improved lower and upper body flexibility (Chen et al., 2008). Gently stretching and moving through various poses can help maintain and even increase your range of motion, making everyday activities easier and more comfortable.
- **Strength and lean muscle building:** Chair yoga can effectively build strength and lean muscle. Research published in the International Journal of Yoga Therapy demonstrated that regular chair yoga can improve muscle strength (Noradechanunt et al., 2017). The resistance provided by your body weight and the chair can help tone muscles.
- **Weight loss:** Chair yoga may not be as intense as other forms of exercise,but it still contributes to weight loss. Women who practiced restorative yoga lost more subcutaneous fat over 48 weeks than those who only stretched (Kanaya et al., 2014). Chair yoga can be an excellent starting point for those beginning their weight loss journey or looking for a low-impact option to complement their existing routine.
- **Effective restorative movements for joint mobility and pain relief:** Chair yoga can offer significant relief for those with joint pain or conditions like arthritis. A randomized controlled trial showed that people who practiced chair yoga experienced reduced pain and improved physical function (Park et al., 2014). The gentle movements and supported poses in chair yoga can help lubricate joints and reduce stiffness without putting excessive stress on sensitive areas.
- **Increased energy:** Chair yoga is reported to increase energy levels and reduce fatigue (Hartfiel. 2012). Combining movement, breathing exercises, and mindfulness in chair yoga can help invigorate your body and mind.
- **Improved balance:** Chair yoga's controlled movements and postures can help strengthen the muscles needed for good balance and increase body awareness.

As with any new exercise program, it's always wise to consult your healthcare provider before starting chair yoga, especially if you have any pre-existing health conditions.

CHAPTER 2

GETTING STARTED—PREPARING FOR YOUR CHAIR YOGA JOURNEY

$\mathcal{B}$eginning your chair yoga journey is an exciting step towards improved health and well-being. This chapter is dedicated to setting up your chair yoga space so that you can gain the most from your workouts. In addition, you'll be introduced to props that can be used to modify each of your poses.

In the following pages, we'll explore the essentials of setting up your practice space, choosing the right chair, and gathering any additional props that might enhance your experience. You'll learn about the importance of proper posture and alignment and basic breathing techniques that form the foundation of any yoga practice.

We'll also discuss setting realistic goals for your chair yoga journey and integrating this practice into your daily routine. Whether you're looking to practice at home, in the office, or even while traveling, we'll provide practical tips to help you make chair yoga a consistent and enjoyable part of your life.

Setting Up a Comfortable Place at Home

Creating a dedicated space for your chair yoga practice can significantly enhance your experience and help you maintain a consistent routine.

- **Floor space:** While chair yoga doesn't require as much space as traditional yoga, it's still important to have enough room to move comfortably. Aim for at least 3 feet by 3 feet around your chair. This will give you ample space to extend your arms and legs without feeling cramped. If you plan to stand occasionally or do poses beside the chair, consider allowing for a bit more space.
- **Floor type:** The ideal floor for chair yoga is flat, stable, and not slippery. Hardwood, tile, or low-pile carpet works well. If you have a slick floor, consider placing a non-slip yoga mat under your chair for added stability. For those with hard floors who want extra cushioning, a thicker yoga mat can provide comfort for any floor-based exercises you incorporate into your routine.

- **Environment:** Your chair yoga space should be a calm, inviting area that encourages relaxation and focus.
- **Lighting:** Natural light is ideal, but if that's not possible, opt for soft, warm lighting that doesn't strain your eyes.
- **Temperature:** Ensure the room is comfortably warm. Consider having a light blanket nearby for relaxation at the end of your practice.
- **Ventilation:** Good air circulation helps keep you fresh and alert during practice. Open a window if weather permits, or use a fan if needed.
- **Minimal distractions:** Choose a quiet area of your home away from high-traffic zones. Practice in a clutter-free space to help maintain mental clarity.

Tips for Stress Relief: Incorporating stress-relieving elements into your chair yoga space can enhance the calming effects of your practice.

- **Aromatherapy:** Use a diffuser with calming essential oils like lavender or chamomile. A study in the Journal of Alternative and Complementary Medicine found that lavender aromatherapy reduced stress and anxiety in patients undergoing dialysis (Gao et al., 2022).
- **Soothing sounds:** Play soft background music or nature sounds. Research published in the Journal of Clinical Nursing showed that music therapy significantly reduced stress in patients with dementia (Lam et al., 2020).
- **Plants:** Add some greenery to your space. A Journal of Physiological Anthropology study found that interacting with indoor plants can reduce psychological and physiological stress (Lee et al., 2015).
- **Personal touches:** Include items that bring you joy or calm, such as family photos, inspirational quotes, or meaningful artwork.
- **Hydration station:** Keep a water bottle nearby to stay hydrated during and after practice.

Keep in mind that your chair yoga space should feel personal and inviting. Experiment with different setups until you find what works best for your needs and preferences. In a comfortable, stress-reducing environment, you'll be more likely to maintain a regular chair yoga practice and reap its many benefits.

Choosing the Right Chair

The appropriate chair is crucial for a safe and effective chair yoga practice. The right chair will provide stability, comfort, and support throughout your sessions.

Ideal types of chairs include:

- Sturdy, straight-backed chairs provide the best support and stability for most chair yoga poses.
- Folding chairs are great for portability, but they should also be sturdy and have a weight capacity that exceeds your body weight.
- Office chairs can work well, especially with adjustable height and locking wheels.

When choosing your chair, you should also consider:

- **Seat height:** Ideally, your feet should rest flat on the floor with your knees at a 90-degree angle. A seat height of 17-19 inches (43-48 cm) works well for most adults.
- **Seat depth:** Aim for a depth that allows you to sit with your back against the backrest while leaving 2-3 inches of space between the edge of the seat and the back of your knees. A depth of 15-18 inches (38-46 cm) is typically suitable.
- **Backrest:** Look for a backrest that supports your lower back. A height of 12-19 inches (30-48 cm) above the seat is generally appropriate.
- **Seat width:** Ensure the seat is wide enough to comfortably accommodate your hips. A width of 20-22 inches (51-56 cm) is usually sufficient for most people.

What Chairs Should Not Be Used

- **Chairs with wheels or casters:** These can be unstable and potentially dangerous during practice.
- **Rocking chairs or recliners:** The movement of these chairs can interfere with balance and stability.
- **Chairs with arms:** While not strictly prohibited, armrests can limit movement in some poses. If your chair has arms, ensure they're low enough not to interfere with your practice.
- **Unstable or rickety chairs:** Any chair that wobbles or feels unsteady should be avoided to prevent accidents.

Good Chairs That Can Be Used

- **Dining room chairs:** Many standard dining chairs offer the right combination of stability and support.
- **Folding metal chairs:** Look for those with rubber feet for added stability. The National Public Seating 9300 Series is a good example, known for its durability and comfort.
- **Wooden kitchen chairs:** These often provide a good balance of comfort and stability. The Winsome Wood Windsor Chair is a popular choice among chair yoga practitioners.
- **Adjustable office chairs:** If using an office chair, opt for one with minimal padding and a straight back, like the HON Exposure Mesh Task Chair. Remember to lock the wheels and height adjustments during practice.

When selecting your chair, always prioritize safety and stability. The best chair for you should feel comfortable and secure and allow you to maintain proper alignment throughout your practice.

Tools and Props for Your Chair Yoga Practice

While chair yoga is designed to be accessible with minimal equipment, incorporating a few carefully chosen props can enhance your practice, providing additional support, comfort, and opportunities for growth.

Yoga Blocks

Yoga blocks can be incredibly versatile in chair yoga. They can help you:

- Elevate your feet if they don't reach the floor
- Provide support for forward bends
- Assist in twists by placing them between your back and the chair

Look for blocks made of foam or cork for comfort and durability.

Yoga Strap or Belt

A yoga strap can help you:

- Extend your reach in seated forward bends
- Assist in shoulder openers
- Aid in leg stretches

Blanket or Towel

A folded blanket or towel can:

- Provide extra cushioning on the seat
- Support your lower back
- Be used as a prop for neck and shoulder releases

Any soft, foldable blanket will do, but yoga-specific blankets like the Yogavni Yoga Blanket are designed for this purpose.

Small Pillow or Cushion

A small pillow can:

- Offer lumbar support
- Elevate your hips for better posture
- Support your head during relaxation

Any small, firm pillow will suffice.

Resistance Bands

Light resistance bands can:

- Add strength training elements to your practice
- Assist in stretches
- Help improve flexibility

In addition to these props, consider downloading a fitness timer that can be set to your required pose lengths. This will ensure you're flowing between poses without pausing for too long.

While props can enhance your practice, they're not necessary. Start with what you have and gradually add props as you see fit. Most importantly, always listen to your body and do not push yourself beyond your limits.

Safety Precautions and Modifications for Different Needs and Abilities

Chair yoga is designed to be accessible to people of various abilities and health conditions. However, practicing safely and making appropriate modifications when necessary is crucial.

General Safety Precautions

1. **Consult your healthcare provider:** Before starting any new exercise program, including chair yoga, consult your doctor, especially if you have chronic health conditions or injuries.
2. **Use a stable chair:** Ensure your chair is sturdy and doesn't wobble. If using a folding chair, check it's fully open and locked.
3. **Proper positioning:** Sit with your feet flat on the floor, back straight, and shoulders relaxed.
4. **Listen to your body:** Stop immediately if a pose causes pain or severe discomfort. Discomfort is normal, but pain is not.
5. **Breathe steadily:** Maintain regular breathing throughout your practice. Never hold your breath during poses.
6. **Stay hydrated:** Keep water nearby and drink as needed.

Modifications for Different Needs

Limited Mobility:

- Use straps or belts to extend your reach in stretches
- Perform twists by holding the chair back instead of your body

Balance Issues:

- Keep one hand on the chair at all times during standing poses
- Use a wall or sturdy furniture for additional support

Arthritis:

- Move slowly and gently, especially in weight-bearing joints
- Use cushions or folded blankets for extra joint support

Back Pain:

- Use a small pillow or rolled towel for lumbar support
- Avoid deep forward bends; instead, focus on gentle back arches

Each exercise in the coming chapters will also provide variations you can use to modify your poses for beginners and options to deepen your stretch.

Finally, before you begin your warm-up movements and poses, remember that everyone's body and needs are different. It's essential to work within your current abilities and honor your body as it becomes stronger, leaner, and healthier.

CHAPTER 3
WARMING-UP

*B*efore you begin with the chair yoga poses that will become the foundation of your weight loss journey, you need to know how to warm up properly.

When your body is at rest, your muscles, cardiovascular system, and joints are preserved. To maximize your calorie burn and prevent injury, it's essential to raise your heart rate slightly, pump oxygen-rich blood to your muscles, and loosen your joints.

In addition, warming up provides you with the unique opportunity to focus on your movements, pay attention to your breath, and begin your workout with intention.

Seated Cat-Cow Stretch

This pose combination improves spinal flexibility and releases back tension.

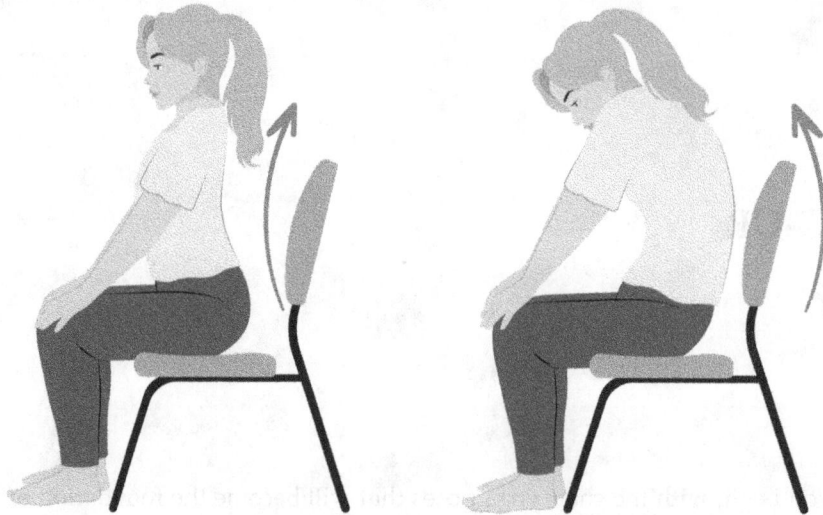

Instructions

- Take your seat, sitting tall in your chair with your feet in front of you, knees together, and feet flat on the floor.
- Rest your hands on your knees, palms down, and gaze forward in a neutral position.
- Focus on your breath and your next conscious inhale. Arch your back and look upwards.
- Allow your shoulders to roll back and lift your chest to open it up. This is your Cow pose.
- Hold your Cow pose for a full breath count, and on your next exhale, round your spine.
- Tuck your chin towards your chest, letting your shoulders roll forward and draw your navel in towards your spine. This is your Cat pose.
- Hold for a full breath count before inhaling again and returning to your Cow pose.
- Alternate between Cow and Cat pose for 30 seconds.

Modifications

- Easier: Perform smaller, gentler movements if you have limited flexibility.
- Harder: Add arm movements—reach forward in Cat, open wide in Cow.
- Props: Use a small cushion for lower back support if needed.

Tips

- Keep movements slow and controlled.
- Let your breath guide each movement.
- Reduce your range of motion if you feel discomfort, especially in your neck.

Neck Rolls

This gentle exercise helps release neck tension and improves neck mobility.

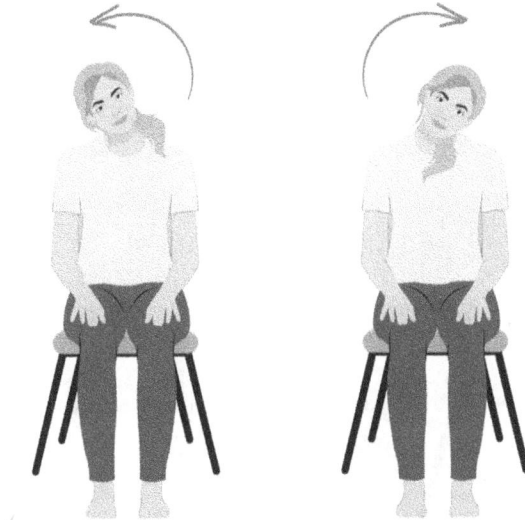

Instructions

- Sit tall in your chair with your feet in front of you, knees together, and feet flat on the floor.
- Rest your hands on your thighs, palms down, and gaze forward in a neutral position.
- Inhale, and as you do, drop your right ear towards your right shoulder.
- Hold this comfortable stretch for 5 seconds.
- On your next inhale, roll your head forward and bring your chin towards your chest.
- Hold for 5 seconds, and on your next inhale, roll your head to the left, bringing your left ear towards your left shoulder.
- Hold this stretch for 5 seconds, and on your next inhale, roll your head back to the center.
- Complete five full rotations before beginning a new counterclockwise cycle, dropping your left ear to your left shoulder.

Modifications

- Easier: Perform smaller, gentler movements if you have neck pain or stiffness.
- Harder: Hold each position for a few breaths before moving to the next.
- Props: Use a small rolled towel behind your neck for support if needed.

Tips

- Move slowly and gently, avoiding any jerky or rapid movements.
- Don't force the stretch; work within your comfortable range of motion.
- If you experience any pain or dizziness, stop the exercise.

Shoulder Rolls

This exercise helps release upper body tension and improves shoulder mobility.

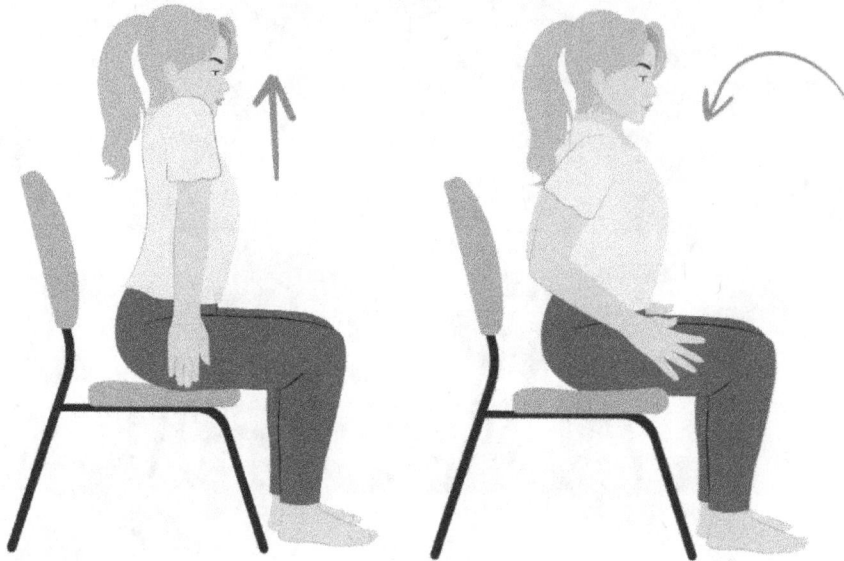

Instructions

- Remain in your seat, sitting tall in your chair with your feet in front of you, knees together, and feet flat on the floor.
- Rest your hands on your thighs, palms down, and gaze forward in a neutral position.
- Focus on your breath and lift your shoulders as you inhale in an exaggerated shrug.
- Hold your shrug for 5 seconds.
- On your next inhale, roll your shoulders back and down, feeling your shoulder blades squeeze together.
- Hold your squeeze position for 5 seconds before returning to a neutral position.
- Continue to shrug and squeeze your shoulders five times.

Modifications

- Easier: Perform smaller movements if you have limited shoulder mobility.
- Harder: Add arm movements, circling your arms as you roll your shoulders.
- Props: None required.

Tips

- Breathe deeply, coordinating your breath with the shoulder movements.
- Focus on releasing tension in your neck and upper back as you roll.
- If you experience any pain or discomfort, reduce the range of motion or stop the exercise.

Seated Side Stretch

This exercise stretches the lateral muscles of the torso, improving flexibility and reducing tension in the sides of the body.

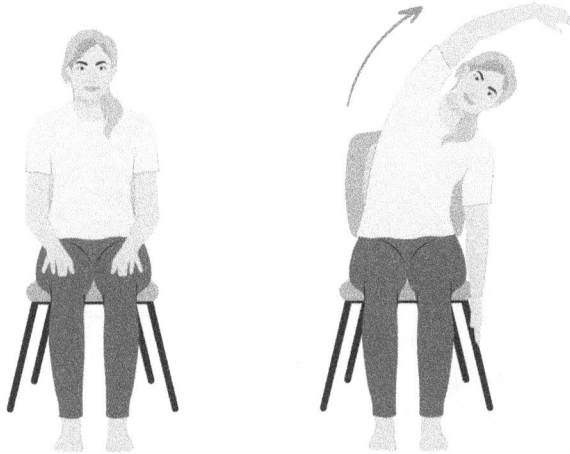

Instructions

- Remain in your seat, sitting tall in your chair with your feet in front of you, knees together, and feet flat on the floor.
- Drop your hands to your sides, resting them alongside your chair, palms facing toward your body.
- Bring focus to your breath, and on your next inhale, reach your right arm toward the ceiling.
- Allow your left hand to slide down the side of the chair.
- Exhale and gently lean to the left, turning your gaze to your right shoulder.
- Hold your stretch for 30 seconds.
- Return to your center and draw focus to your breath once more.
- On your next inhale, reach your left hand towards the ceiling, holding your stretch for 15 seconds.

Modifications

- Easier: Reduce the range of motion, leaning only as far as comfortable.
- Harder: Extend both arms overhead before leaning to each side.
- Props: Use the chair back for support if needed.

Tips

- Keep your sitting bones firmly planted on the chair.
- Avoid twisting your torso; focus on a pure side bend.

Seated Forward Fold with Arms Extended

This pose stretches the back, hamstrings, shoulders, and arms, promoting flexibility and relaxation.

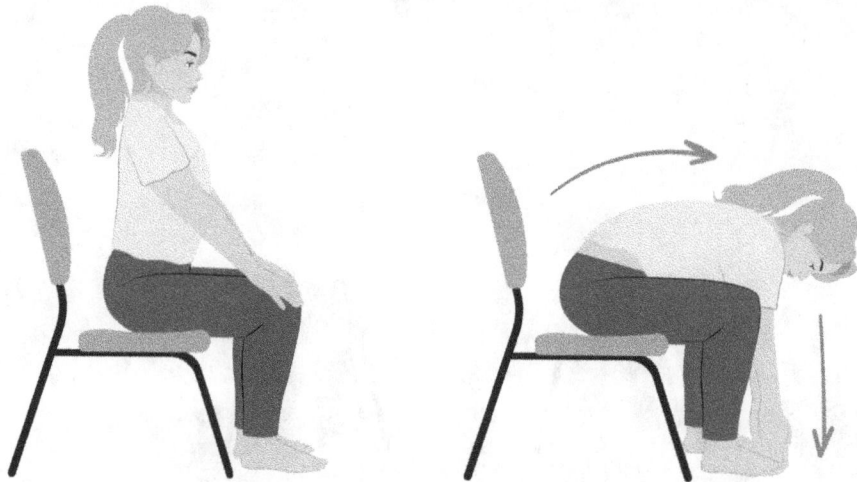

Instructions

- Remain in your seat, sitting tall in your chair with your feet in front of you, your knees slightly less than shoulder-width apart, and your feet flat on the floor.
- Rest your hands on your thighs, palms down, and gaze forward in a neutral position.
- Draw focus to your breath and begin to hinge forward at your hips, slowly sliding your hands down toward the floor.
- On your next exhale, consciously relax your shoulders and head, hanging like a ragdoll.
- Let your hands hang loosely on the floor, and your head hang between your legs if you can.
- Hold your pose for 30 seconds.
- To return to your center, inhale deeply, hinge at your hips, and return to a seated position.

Modifications

- Easier: Sit further forward in your chair to reduce hamstring stretch.
- Harder: Reach for your toes or ankles if flexibility allows.
- Props: Place a cushion on your lap to rest your forehead if needed.

Tips

- Keep your back straight as you hinge forward from the hips.
- Breathe deeply, focusing on releasing tension with each exhale.
- If you feel any strain in your lower back, bend your knees more or come out of the pose.

Short Warm-Up Routine

This quick routine helps prepare your body for further practice by releasing tension in your back, sides, and shoulders.

1. Seated Cat-Cow Stretch: 30 seconds
2. Seated Side Stretch: 30 seconds on each side
3. Seated Forward Fold with Arms Extended: 30 seconds

Remember to breathe deeply throughout the routine and move slowly and mindfully. If you feel any pain or discomfort, ease off the stretch or stop altogether.

Full Warm-Up Routine

This comprehensive warm-up routine prepares your body for a full chair yoga session by targeting key areas: the spine, neck, shoulders, sides, and back.

1. Seated Cat-Cow Stretch: 30 seconds
2. Neck Rolls: 1 minute on each side
3. Shoulder rolls: 15 seconds on each side
4. Seated Side Stretch: 30 seconds on each side
5. Seated Forward Fold with Extended Arms: 30 seconds

Breathing Techniques

Breathing is an unconscious act that can profoundly affect your body when consciously harnessed. When you are stressed or anxious, your breathing becomes shallow and rapid, which can lead to even more stress and anxiety.

When you use conscious, mindful breathing techniques, you send a signal to your nervous system, encouraging your parasympathetic nervous system to activate. This system is directly responsible for your rest and digest function, which helps combat stress, heal your body, and aid in weight loss.

Each breathing exercise below can be used as a stand-alone practice or as part of your chair yoga routine to maximize calorie burn during workouts.

Diaphragmatic Breathing

This is belly breathing, and you can call it that. This technique focuses on your diaphragm (the dome-shaped muscle at the base of your lungs).

1. On your chair, take a slow, deep breath through your nose and feel your belly expand.
2. Then, exhale slowly through your mouth and feel your belly deflate.
3. Do this for a few minutes, and just focus on the rising and deflating of your belly.

This breathing technique can help you reduce stress and anxiety, improve digestion, and lower your blood pressure.

Mindful Breathing

Mindful breathing is excellent for increasing your inner calmness and bringing clarity to your thoughts.

1. While sitting on your chair, close your eyes and take a few deep breaths.
2. Here, you will inhale through your nose and exhale through your mouth. Allow yourself to settle into the moment and let go of any thoughts.
3. Then, focus on the sensation of your breath moving in and out of your body. You will notice the air entering your nostrils and filling your lungs.
4. Your mind will wander at some point, but that's normal; just let it go. If your mind starts following a thought, return it to your breath.
5. Just do this until you start feeling more relaxed.

Access to Instructional Videos

Thank you for choosing my book!
Enjoy exclusive access to instructional videos for every pose in the 28-day program by scanning the QR code below with your phone camera.
A link will appear. Tap the link, and it will take you to the videos.

https://youtube.com/playlist?list=PLCmP4fdibl_S1_dcOXZwUrG25dTGRJAcu&si=VqYXL1qldMT_L0h0

CHAPTER 4
WEEK 1—GENTLE BEGINNINGS

*a*s you begin your first week of chair yoga, you may feel excitement, anticipation, or even slight trepidation. All of these emotions are normal. The best way to build consistency and incorporate anything new into your life is to integrate it into existing routines. With this in mind, let's examine some daily routines that allow you to integrate your 10-minute chair yoga workouts.

Morning

Morning workouts before your coffee or tea can help you ease into the day, energize yourself, and provide a healthy boost of dopamine, the hormone that induces feelings of happiness. Select your short warm-up and one of the routines listed below based on your fitness, flexibility, or strength levels.

Midday

Midday routines allow you to break the monotony of the day, reenergize as you approach the typical midday slump, and destress. Midday routines are a great time to incorporate one of your breathing exercises, a short warm-up routine, and one of your workout routines based on your fitness, flexibility, or strength levels.

Evening

Completing your chair yoga workout in the evening will allow you to end your day by releasing pent-up stress and energy and providing your body with an extra boost of relaxation as you enter into a natural state of rest and digest. Each of the routines provided is at most 10 minutes long, but feel free to add your favorite chair yoga poses at the end of every routine.

Finally, always remember that consistency is your most powerful weight-loss weapon. Whether in your diet, managing stress, getting enough quality sleep, or working out, taking small steps every day toward positive change will result in you achieving your goals.

Day 1-4: Basic Chair Yoga Poses for Beginners

Your foundational chair yoga poses are beginner-friendly and allow you to lose weight effectively. Each pose will give you the strength you need to use more advanced poses. As you enter this first set of poses, focus on the correctness of each pose, engage your muscles, and work with your breath.

Seated Mountain Pose

This foundational pose promotes proper alignment, improves posture, and centers the body and mind. Ensuring your mountain pose is correct is critical, as it is the foundational pose for all other poses and movements.

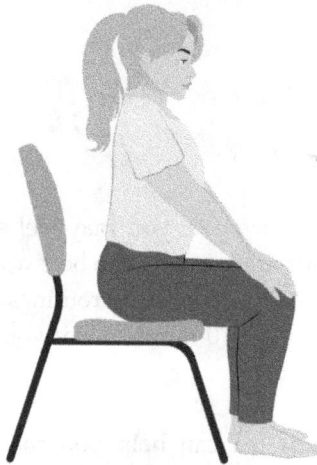

Instructions

- Take your seat, sitting tall in your chair with your feet in front of you, knees together, and feet flat on the floor.
- Rest your hands on your knees, palms down, and gaze forward in a neutral position.
- Inhale deeply, and as you exhale, press into your sitting bones and lengthen your spine.
- As you inhale, engage your core, roll your shoulders back and down, and lift your chest.
- Remain in your mountain pose for 1 minute.

Modifications

- Easier: Use a chair with back support if needed.
- Harder: Close your eyes to increase body awareness.
- Props: Place a folded blanket under your feet if they don't reach the floor.

Tips

- Relax your face and jaw while maintaining the posture.

Chair Forward Fold

This pose stretches the back, hamstrings, and calves while promoting relaxation and improved circulation to the head.

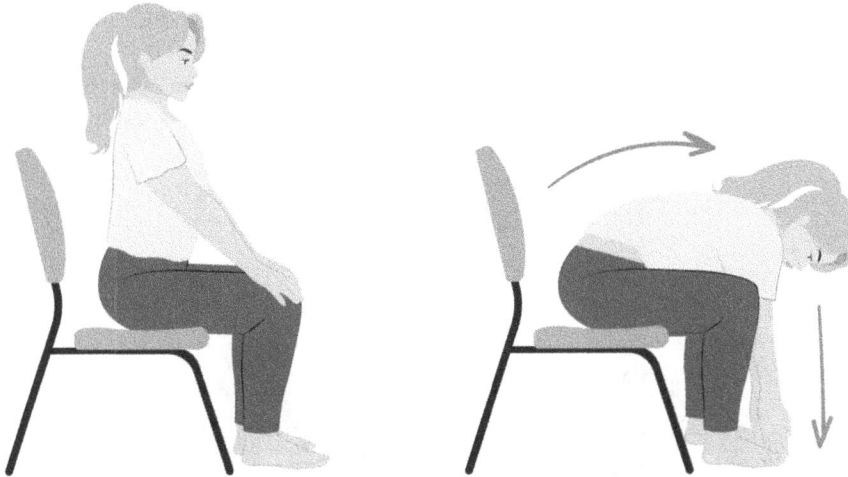

Instructions

- Begin in your neutral mountain pose, feet flat on the floor and your hands on your thighs.
- Draw focus to your breath, and as you inhale, open your legs slightly wider than hip-width apart.
- Ensure your toes are facing forward and your spine is straight.
- As you exhale, slowly lower your upper body between your knees. Keep your spine straight and your behind firmly planted on the seat.
- Inhale and clasp your hands together. Slowly straighten your legs to a comfortable stretch without adjusting your upper body.
- Remain in your pose for 1 minute.
- To return to your centered position, sit up by hinging at your hips, bend your knees and bring them together, and place your hands on your thighs.

Modifications

- Easier: Keep knees bent if hamstrings are tight.
- Harder: Reach for your ankles or feet if flexibility allows.
- Props: Rest your forearms on a yoga block placed between your legs.

Tips

- Keep your back straight as you fold forward; hinge from the hips.
- Don't force your body into the stretch; go only as far as is comfortable.
- If you feel any strain in your lower back, bend your knees more or come out of the pose.

Seated Side Bend

This pose stretches the lateral muscles of the torso, improving flexibility and posture.

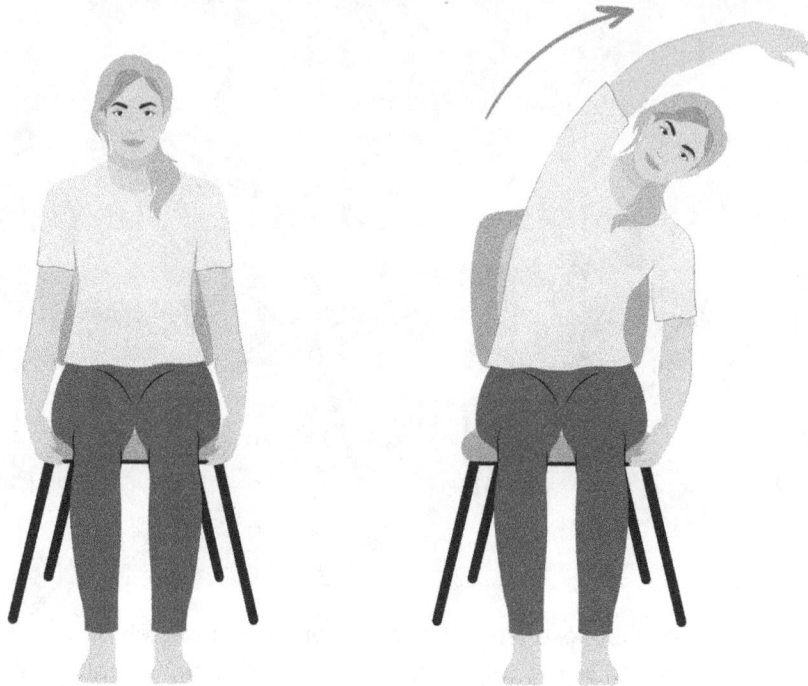

Instructions

- Begin in the mountain pose with your hands at your sides, grasping the seat of your chair.
- Inhale deeply and sweep your right arm toward the ceiling, palm facing out and up.
- Exhale, and as you do, lean to the left, bend your left elbow, and stretch your right side.
- Draw focus to your breath and hold the pose for 30 seconds.
- Return to your center and complete the pose on the other side.
- Once complete, return to your mountain pose.

Modifications

- Easier: Reduce the range of motion, leaning only as far as comfortable.
- Harder: Extend both arms overhead before leaning to each side.
- Props: Use the chair seat for support with your lower hand if needed.

Tips

- Keep your sitting bones firmly planted on the chair.
- Avoid twisting your torso; focus on a pure side bend, breathing deeply.
- If you feel pain, especially in your lower back, reduce the stretch or stop.

Seated Twist

This pose improves spinal mobility, relieves back tension, and can aid digestion.

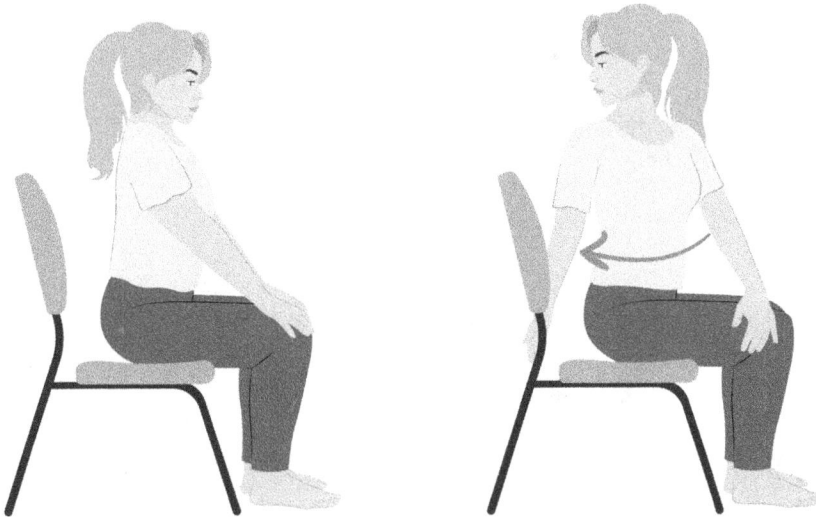

Instructions

- Remain seated in a neutral mountain pose.
- Bring focus to your breath and place your hands at your sides next to your thighs.
- As you exhale, twist your upper body to the right, ensuring your sit bones remain on the chair.
- Bring your right hand to the back of the chair and your left hand to your right knee.
- Focus on your breath once more and hold your pose for 30 seconds.
- On your next inhale, release your pose and return to your neutral seated position.
- Repeat your pose on the other side for 30 seconds.

Modifications

- Easier: Keep both hands on your knees if reaching the chair back is uncomfortable.
- Harder: Look over your shoulder to deepen the twist.
- Props: Use a chair with a back for support.

Tips

- Keep your sit bones firmly planted on the chair as you twist.
- Twist from your mid-back, not your lower back.
- If you feel pain, especially in your lower back, reduce the twist or stop.

Seated Eagle Arms

This pose stretches the upper back and shoulders, alleviating tension and improving arm mobility.

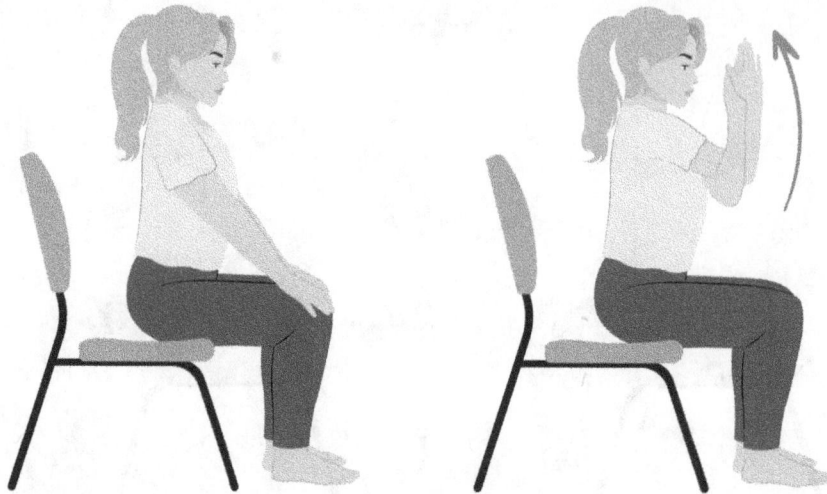

Instructions

- From your mountain pose, sit forward slightly so your behind is about midway in your seat.
- Inhale deeply and bring your arms out to your side so that they are parallel to the floor.
- As you exhale, bring your arms forward, crossing your right arm over your left.
- Bring the outsides of your hands together if you can and ensure your elbows remain in contact.
- Hold your pose for 30 seconds before releasing and returning to your starting position.
- Repeat your pose on the other side before returning to the mountain pose.

Modifications

- Easier: Simply cross your arms in front of your chest if bringing hands together is uncomfortable.
- Harder: Lift your elbows slightly while maintaining the arm position to deepen the stretch.
- Props: None required.

Tips

- Keep your shoulders relaxed and away from your ears, focusing on spreading your shoulder blades as you hold the pose.
- If you feel any shoulder or elbow pain, release the pose immediately.
- Breathe deeply, imagining tension releasing from your upper back with each exhale.

Chair Tree Pose

This pose improves balance and focus.

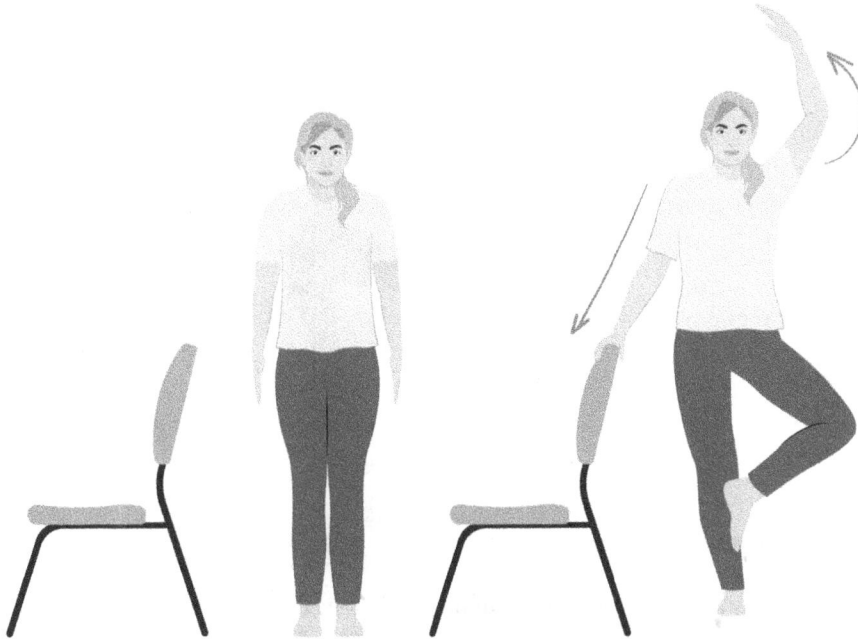

Instructions

- Move your position to the back of your chair and stand with your right side to the backrest.
- Place your right hand on the backrest, inhale, lift your left foot off the floor and engage your core.
- Place the sole of your foot on your calf. Do *not* place your foot on your knee.
- Draw focus to your breath and as you inhale, sweep your left arm up toward the ceiling.
- Keep your elbow slightly bent and your palm facing the ground.
- Gaze forward and hold your pose for 30 seconds.
- Return your left leg to the floor and turn around so your left side faces the backrest.
- Repeat your pose on the other side.

Modifications

- Easier: Keep the raised foot on the ankle instead of the calf.
- Harder: Gaze upward at raised hand.
- Props: Use the chair back for support.

Tips

- Keep your standing leg straight but not locked.
- If you feel unsteady, focus on a fixed point.

Chair Dancer Pose

This pose improves balance, stretches the front body, and strengthens the legs and back.

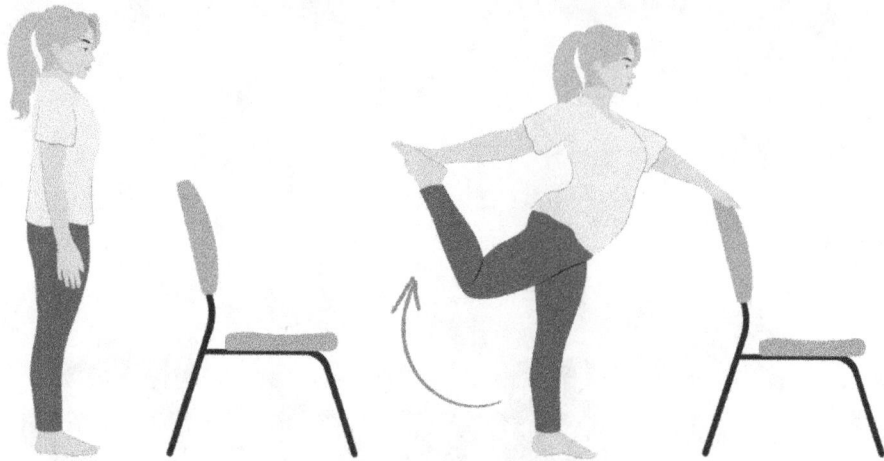

Instructions

- Stand facing your chair's backrest about half an arm's length from the chair.
- Place your hands on the backrest and stand up straight with your toes facing forward.
- Inhale, and as you do, lift your left leg off the floor.
- Bend your knee and push your leg back.
- Exhale and move your left hand off the chair, reaching back to grab your left foot.
- Hold your pose for 30 seconds.
- Return your left leg to the floor and your left arm to the chair.
- Inhale, lift your right leg off the floor, and repeat the pose on the other side.

Modifications

- Easier: Keep both hands on the chair backrest for balance.
- Harder: Let go of the chair with both hands, balancing independently.
- Props: Chair.

Tips

- Keep the standing leg slightly bent to protect the knee.
- Engage your core for stability, focusing on lifting your chest as you bend back.
- If the balance is challenging, fix your gaze on a steady point.

Seated Bound Angle Pose

This pose opens the hips, stretches the inner thighs, and promotes relaxation.

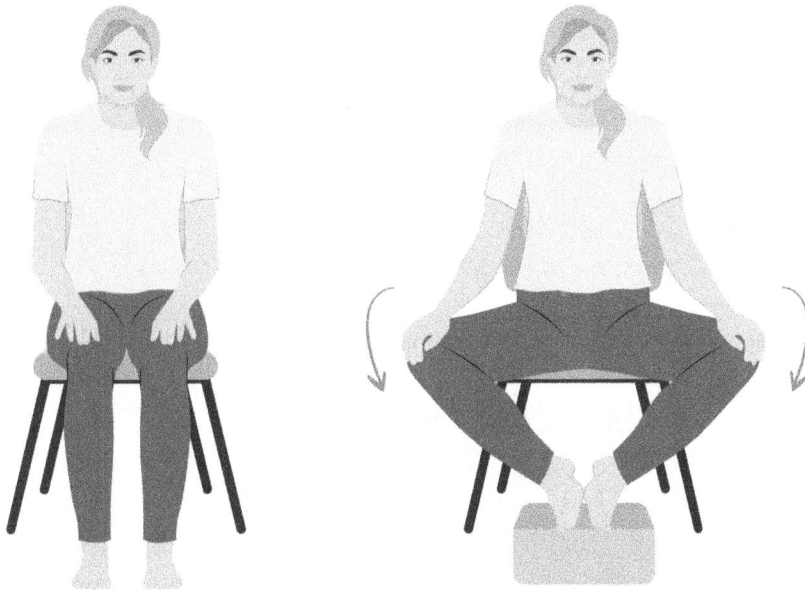

Instructions

- Begin in your neutral mountain pose, feet flat on the floor and your hands on your thighs.
- Inhale and lengthen your spine, fixing your gaze on a point straight in front of you.
- Exhale and bring the soles of your feet together.
- Allow your knees to fall out to the sides.
- Inhale once more and move your hands to the insides of your thighs.
- Engage your core and press your hands into your thighs to deepen your stretch.
- Hold your pose for 1 minute.
- To release your pose, return your hands to the tops of your thighs and place your feet on the floor.
- Bring your knees together to enter the mountain pose.

Modifications

- Easier: Place cushions under the outer thighs for support.
- Harder: Fold forward from hips, reaching for your feet.
- Props: Use blocks under knees if hips are tight.

Tips

- Don't force your knees down; let gravity do the work.
- Keep your spine straight, with your sit bones grounded.
- Focus on breathing into any areas of tension.

Chair Yoga for Weight Loss: Day 1 to 4

Warm-up: 2 minutes

1. Seated Mountain Pose: 1 minute
2. Seated Forward Fold: 1 minute
3. Seated Side Bend: 30 seconds on each side
4. Seated Twist: 30 seconds on each side
5. Seated Eagle Arms: 30 seconds on each side
6. Chair Tree Pose: 1 minute
7. Chair Dancer Pose: 30 seconds on each side
8. Seated Bound Angle: 1 minute

Remember to move slowly and mindfully between poses, listen to your body, and adjust as needed. If any pose causes discomfort, modify or skip it. Breathe deeply throughout the routine, using your breath to guide your movements and deepen your practice.

Day 5-7: Chair Yoga Poses

Five-Pointed Star

This pose strengthens the legs, opens the chest, and improves overall body awareness.

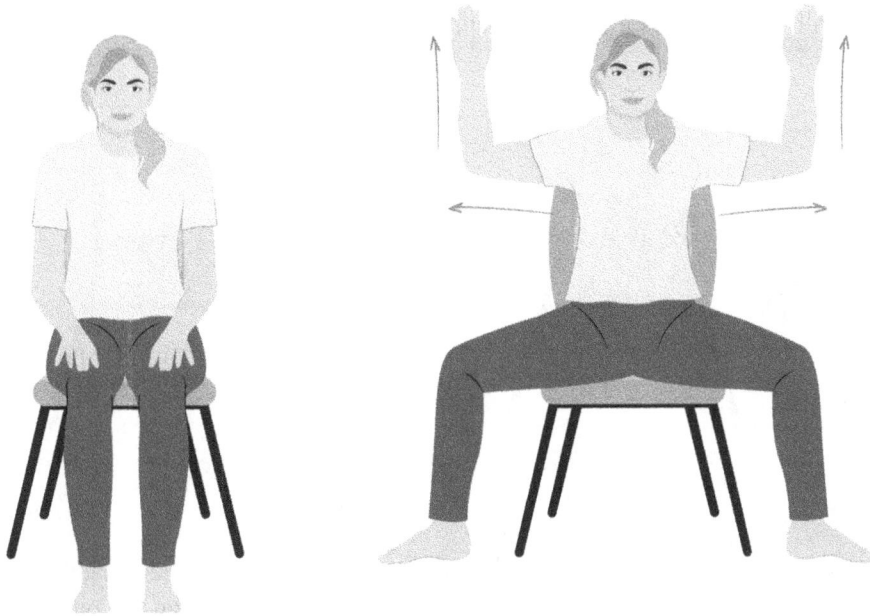

<u>Instructions</u>

- Begin in your neutral mountain pose, feet flat on the floor and your hands on your thighs.
- Inhale and open your legs, widening them to more than hip-width apart.
- Point your toes out at a 45-degree angle and lengthen your spine.
- Inhale and sweep your arms out to your sides. Keep your elbows straight and your palms facing away from your body.
- Exhale and bend your arms. Spread your fingers wide. Inhale and engage your core.
- Exhale and drop your shoulders back into a relaxed position.
- Hold your pose for 1 minute.

<u>Modifications</u>

- Easier: Keep arms lower if shoulder mobility is limited.
- Harder: Lift heels off the floor, balancing on toes.
- Props: Use the chair back for support if balance is challenging.

<u>Tips</u>

- Keep your spine straight and chest open throughout the pose.

Seated Cat-Cow Stretch

This pose combination improves spinal flexibility and releases back tension.

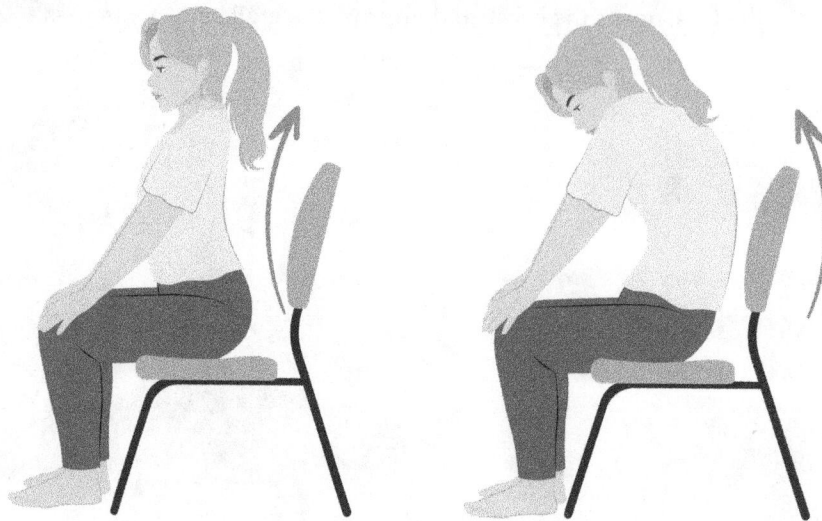

Instructions

- Take your seat, sitting tall in your chair with your feet in front of you, knees together, and feet flat on the floor.
- Rest your hands on your knees, palms down, and gaze forward in a neutral position.
- Focus on your breath and your next conscious inhale. Arch your back and look upwards.
- Allow your shoulders to roll back and lift your chest to open it up. This is your Cow pose.
- Hold your Cow pose for a full breath count, and on your next exhale, round your spine.
- Tuck your chin towards your chest, letting your shoulders roll forward and draw your navel in towards your spine. This is your Cat pose.
- Hold for a full breath count, before inhaling again and returning to your Cow pose.
- Alternate between Cow and Cat pose for 1 minute.

Modifications

- Easier: Perform smaller, gentler movements if you have limited flexibility.
- Harder: Add arm movements—reach forward in Cat, open wide in Cow.
- Props: Use a small cushion for lower back support if needed.

Tips

- Keep movements slow and controlled, focusing on the stretch and release in your spine.
- Let your breath guide each movement.
- Reduce your range of motion if you feel discomfort, especially in your neck.

Seated Twist

This pose improves spinal mobility, relieves back tension, and can aid digestion.

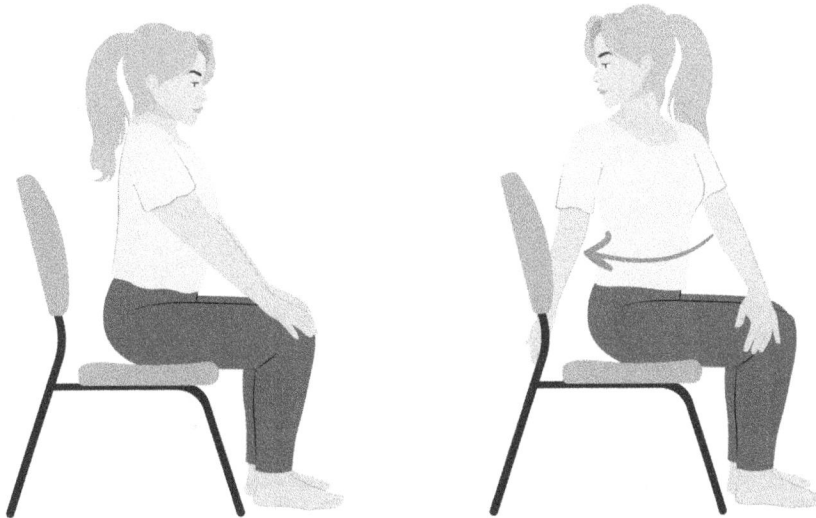

<u>Instructions</u>

- Remain seated in a neutral mountain pose.
- Bring focus to your breath and place your hands at your sides next to your thighs.
- As you exhale, twist your upper body to the right, ensuring your sit bones remain on the chair.
- Bring your right hand to the back of the chair and your left hand to your right knee.
- Focus on your breath once more and hold your pose for 30 seconds.
- On your next inhale, release your pose and return to your neutral seated position.
- Repeat your pose on the other side for 30 seconds.

<u>Modifications</u>

- Easier: Keep both hands on your knees if reaching the chair back is uncomfortable.
- Harder: Look over your back shoulder to deepen the twist.
- Props: Use a chair with a back for support.

<u>Tips</u>

- Keep your sit bones firmly planted on the chair as you twist.
- Twist from your mid-back, not your lower back.
- If you feel pain, especially in your lower back, reduce the twist or stop.

Chair Extended Triangle Pose

This pose strengthens the legs, stretches the sides of the torso, and improves balance. You may need an extra chair or a sturdy piece of furniture for this pose.

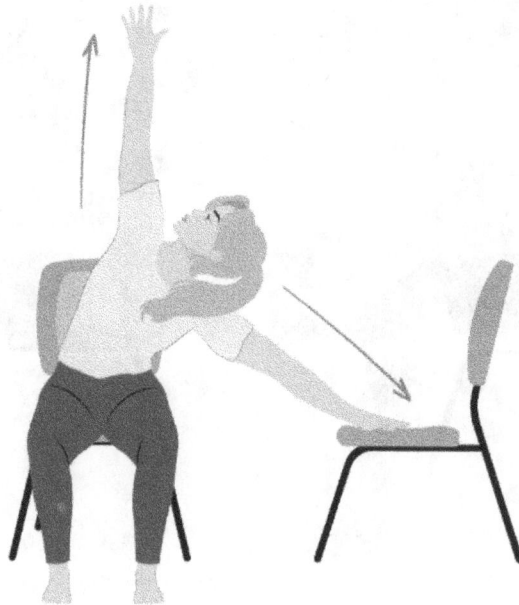

Instructions

- Begin in your neutral mountain pose, feet flat on the floor and your hands on your thighs.
- Your second chair should be on your right side.
- Inhale and sweep your hands up above your head.
- Exhale, and lean to the right, allowing your right hand to rest on the chair next to you.
- Gaze up toward your left hand and hold your pose for 30 seconds.
- Return to an upright position, drop your arms, and switch to your other chair.
- Inhale and sweep your hands up, repeating your pose on the other side.

Modifications

- Easier: Place your hand higher on the chair back instead of the seat.
- Harder: Extend the top arm straight up towards the ceiling.
- Props: Second chair or sturdy furniture piece.

Tips

- Align shoulders over hips as much as possible and breathe deeply, focusing on the stretch in your side body.
- If you feel any strain in your lower back, bend your front knee slightly.

Seated Leg Extension

This pose stretches the hamstrings and calves, promoting circulation in the legs and knees.

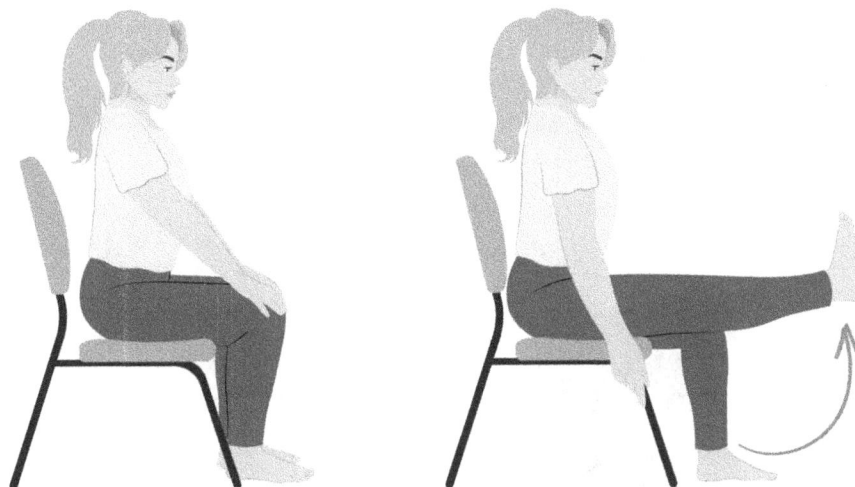

Instructions

- From your mountain pose, sit forward slightly so your behind is about midway in your seat.
- Drop your arms to your sides and hold on to the seating area of your chair.
- Inhale, and as you do, lift your right leg straight out in front of you.
- Keep your foot flexed and your spine straight. Ensure your gaze is forward.
- Hold your pose for 30 seconds.
- Release your pose by bending your right knee and placing it back on the floor.
- Repeat your pose on the other side before returning to the mountain pose.

Modifications

- Easier: Keep a slight bend in your knee if the hamstring stretch is too intense.
- Harder: Reach for your toes with your hands if flexibility allows.
- Props: Use a strap around your foot to assist with the stretch if needed.

Tips

- Keep your spine straight and avoid rounding your back.
- Engage your quadriceps to deepen the hamstring stretch.
- If you feel knee or lower back pain, reduce the extension or stop.

Seated Knee to Chest Stretch

This pose stretches the lower back, hips, and glutes, promoting relaxation and relieving lower body tension.

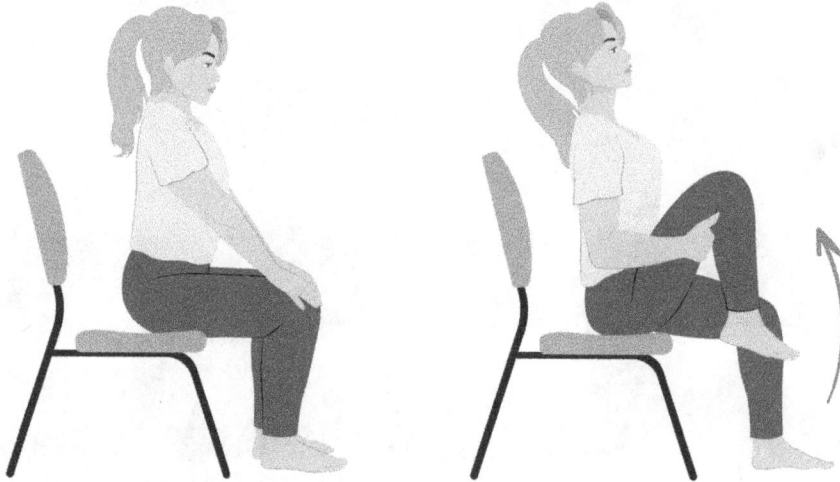

Instructions

- From your mountain pose, sit forward slightly so your behind is about midway in your seat.
- Inhale deeply, and as you do, lift your right foot off the floor.
- Interlace your fingers under your thigh, and as you exhale, draw your right knee closer to your chest.
- Ensure your spine is straight and long and that your gaze is forward.
- Hold your pose for 30 seconds.
- Release by gently lowering your foot to the floor and placing your hands on your thighs.
- Repeat the pose on the other side before returning to your mountain pose.

Modifications

- Easier: Use your hands to support your thigh instead of interlacing fingers if reaching is difficult.
- Harder: Extend your opposite leg straight while holding your knee to your chest.
- Props: Use a strap around your thigh if reaching your leg is challenging.

Tips

- Keep your spine straight, and your shoulders relaxed.
- Avoid rounding your back; focus on hinging at the hips.
- If you feel any knee or lower back pain, reduce the stretch or stop.

Chair Warrior III Pose

This pose strengthens the back and improves balance.

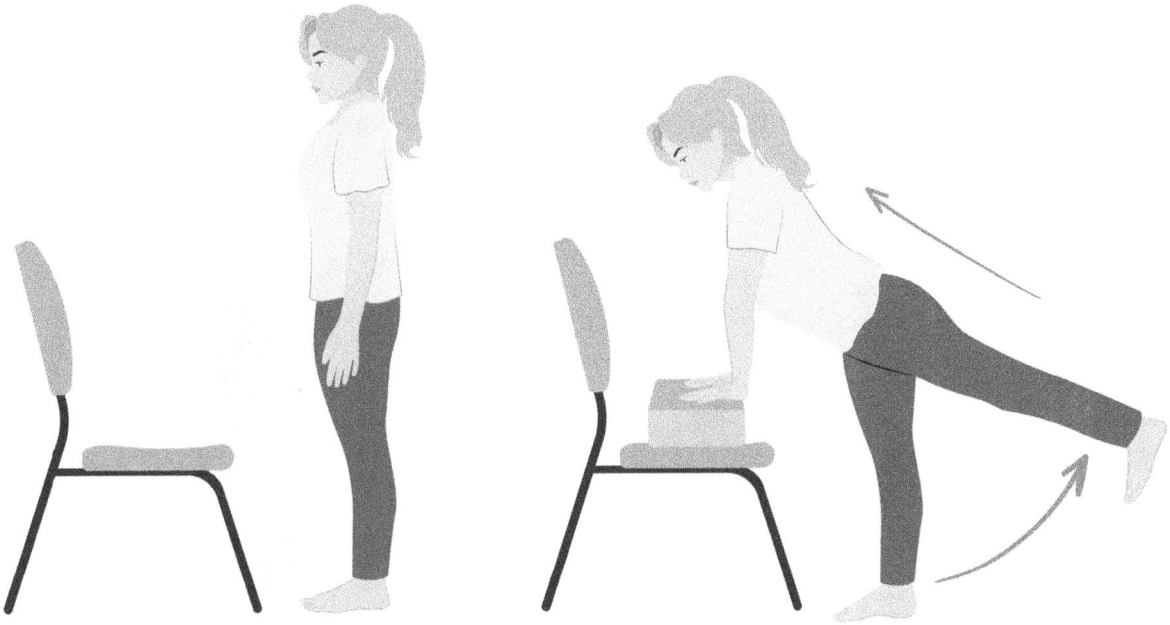

Instructions

- Move to the front of your chair so your body faces the seating area.
- Bring your feet close to the chair and stand tall.
- Inhale, and as you do, lift your right leg off the floor while hinging forward at the hips.
- Drop your hands to the seating area while maintaining a straight line with your spine, and use your right leg for leverage. Gaze down to your hands.
- Hold your pose for 30 seconds.
- Return your right leg to the floor and stand upright.
- Inhale and lift your left leg off the floor to repeat your pose on the other side.

Modifications

- Easier: Keep the standing leg slightly bent.
- Harder: Lift arms parallel to the floor.
- Props: Use blocks on the seat for hand support.

Tips

- Keep hips level throughout the pose.
- Engage core and back muscles.
- Breathe steadily, focusing on balance and alignment.

Seated Eagle Arms

This pose stretches the upper back and shoulders, alleviating tension and improving arm circulation.

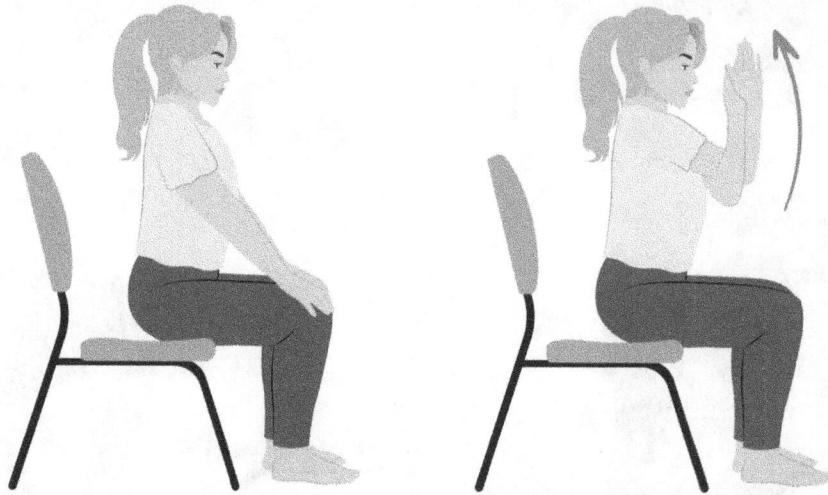

Instructions

- From your mountain pose, sit forward slightly so your behind is about midway in your seat.
- Inhale deeply and bring your arms out to your side so that they are parallel to the floor.
- As you exhale, bring your arms forward, crossing your right arm over your left.
- Bring the outsides of your hands together if you can and ensure your elbows remain in contact.
- Hold your pose for 30 seconds before releasing and returning to your starting position.
- Repeat your pose on the other side before returning to the mountain pose.

Modifications

- Easier: Simply cross your arms in front of your chest if bringing hands together is uncomfortable.
- Harder: Lift your elbows slightly while maintaining the arm position to deepen the stretch.
- Props: None required.

Tips

- Keep your shoulders relaxed and away from your ears.
- Focus on spreading your shoulder blades as you hold the pose.
- If you feel any shoulder or elbow pain, release the pose immediately.

Chair Yoga for Weight Loss: Day 5 to 7

Warm-up: 2 minutes

1. Seated Five-Pointed Star: 1 minute
2. Seated Cat-Cow Stretch: 1 minute
3. Seated Twist: 30 seconds on each side
4. Extended Triangle: 30 seconds on each side
5. Leg Extension: 30 seconds on each side
6. Seated Knee to Chest: 30 seconds on each side
7. Chair Warrior III: 30 seconds on each side
8. Seated Eagle Arms: 30 seconds on each side

Exploring Body Sensations

With your first week complete, you may find that your body is already beginning to feel stronger and that your posture is better. This is perfectly fine if you have yet to see the scale move. While your ultimate goal may be to lose weight, these early phases of your chair yoga journey are designed to build enough strength and endurance for the coming weeks.

Progressive Muscle Relaxation

This is an excellent technique for releasing tension and promoting relaxation. It involves systematically tensing and relaxing different muscle groups throughout the body.

1. On your chair, take a few deep breaths until you begin to relax.
2. Then, starting with your feet, tense all the muscles in your feet and toes and hold that tension for a few seconds.
3. Release the tension, and you will feel your feet and toes relaxing.
4. Move up to your calves, and again, tense all the muscles on your lower legs before releasing them.
5. Continue to go up your body and tense and relax each muscle group in turn: your thighs, hips, belly, chest, arms, hands, neck, and face.

This is an excellent technique for releasing physical tension and increasing a deep sense of relaxation throughout the body.

CHAPTER 5
WEEK 2—BUILDING STRENGTH AND FLEXIBILITY

*W*eek 2 of your 28-day chair yoga regime has some progression, including using the chair as support during standing poses. While basic poses are mostly seated, these new poses will help you develop your stabilizer muscles, allowing your body to grow in strength and flexibility.

Science shows that the lean muscle developed in exercises like chair yoga helps to increase resting metabolism (Thomas & Burns, 2016). With new challenges, however, come feelings of fear and intimidation. To overcome this fear, setting actionable goals for the week is important.

These goals include squeezing in an extra workout for the week, focusing on your water intake, or changing just one unhealthy meal a day to a healthy one. Whatever your goal is for yourself this week, remember that your chair yoga workout doesn't need to be a source of fear. Instead, view your progression as something to be celebrated as your body grows in strength—even if the scale hasn't moved yet.

Strength and Flexibility Poses

This week introduces you to standing chair yoga poses, and as you progress from seated to standing, it's essential to focus on your safety. If you have not yet created a space where your chair is stable, now is the time. Feel free to use props to adapt your poses if you feel unstable or unable to complete the pose correctly, and remember, your poses should never hurt your body. If you experience pain, repeat week 1 so your body can adapt. Alternatively, complete poses from this week that do not hurt and return to more challenging poses once you have gained the strength.

Day 8-11: Chair Yoga Poses

Seated Mountain Pose

This foundational pose promotes proper alignment, improves posture, and centers the body and mind.

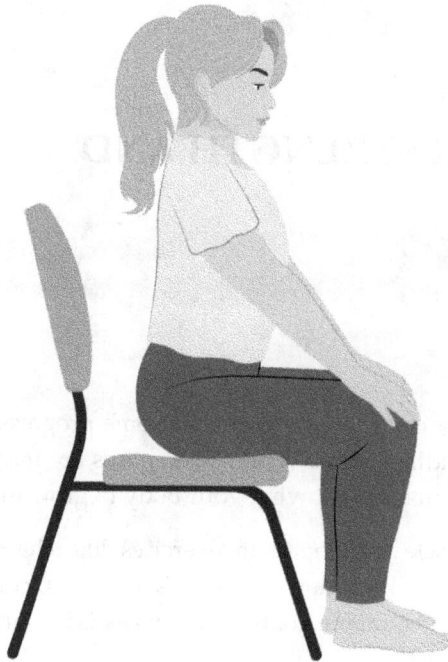

Instructions

- Sit tall in your chair with your feet in front of you, and feet flat on the floor.
- Rest your hands on your knees, palms down, and gaze forward in a neutral position.
- Inhale deeply, and as you exhale, press down into your sitting bones and lengthen your spine.
- As you inhale, engage your core, roll your shoulders back and down, and lift your chest.
- Remain in your mountain pose for 1 minute.

Modifications

- Easier: Use a chair with back support if needed.
- Harder: Close your eyes to increase body awareness.
- Props: Place a folded blanket under your feet if they don't reach the floor.

Tips

- Relax your face and jaw while maintaining the posture.

Seated Forward Bend

This pose stretches the hamstrings, lower back, and calves while promoting relaxation.

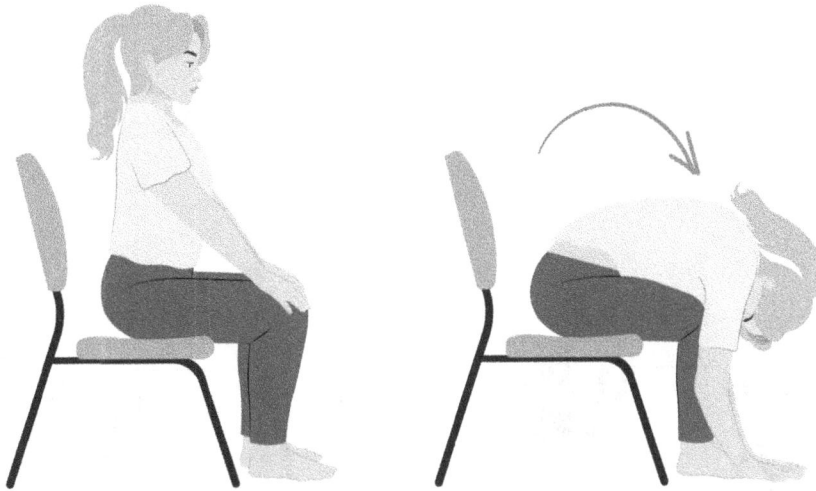

Instructions

- Begin in your neutral mountain pose.
- Inhale and shift forward on your seat, ensuring your feet are flat on the floor and you are comfortably balanced on the front edge of your chair.
- Exhale, and on your next inhale, reach your arms up overhead.
- As you exhale, hinge forward at the hips and lower your torso towards your thighs.
- Allow your arms to dangle towards the floor, and let your head hang heavy.
- Hold your pose for 1 minute, as you will feel your spine lengthening.
- To come out of your pose, inhale, hinge at the hips, and slowly return to an upright position.

Modifications

- Easier: Bend your knees slightly to reduce hamstring stretch.
- Harder: Reach for your ankles or toes if flexibility allows.
- Props: Rest your forearms on a cushion placed on your lap for support.

Tips

- Keep your back straight as you hinge forward from the hips.
- Allow your upper body to relax and hang heavily.
- If you feel any strain in your lower back, bend your knees more or come out of the pose.

Seated Spinal Twist

This pose enhances spinal mobility, relieves back tension, and can aid digestion.

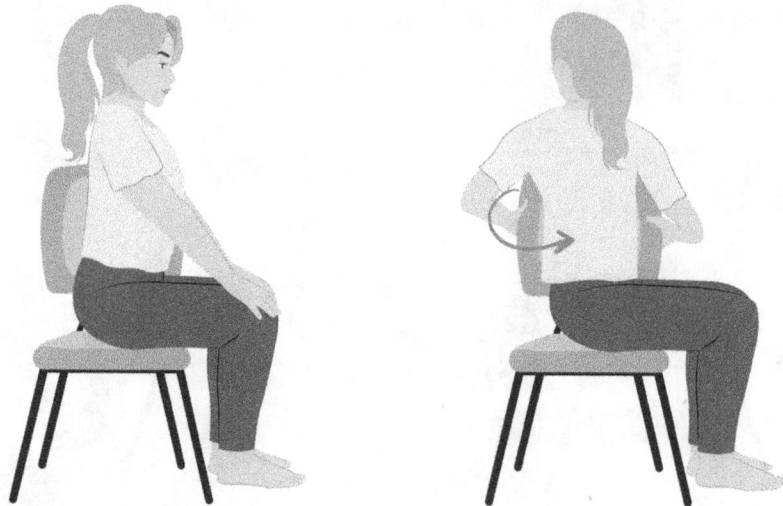

The spinal twist activates your parasympathetic nervous system by stimulating the PSOAS (a pair of large muscles that run from the lumbar spine through the groin on either side).

Instructions

- Turn sideways in your chair, resting your feet flat on the floor.
- Place the hand closest to the backrest on the seat and your other hand on your thigh.
- Inhale, drop your shoulders back, and turn your gaze to the backrest.
- Exhale and twist your upper torso toward the backrest.
- Place both hands on the backrest and guide your upper body to face the backrest while your hips and feet remain in their starting position.
- Hold your pose for 30 seconds.
- Turn around so your other side is against the backrest, and repeat on the other side.

Modifications

- Easier: Keep one hand on the seat if reaching the backrest is uncomfortable.
- Harder: Deepen the twist by looking over your back shoulder.
- Props: Use a chair with a sturdy backrest for support.

Tips

- Move slowly and mindfully into the twist.
- Keep your hips square to the side of the chair and twist from your mid-back, not your lower back.

Seated Figure Four Stretch

This pose targets the glutes, hips, and piriformis muscles, improving flexibility and reducing lower body tension.

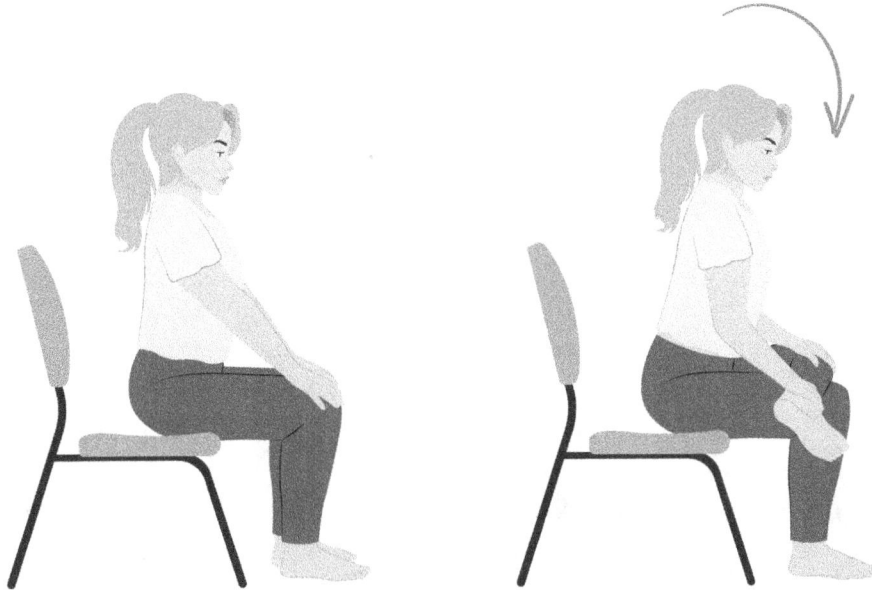

Instructions

- From your mountain pose, sit forward slightly so your behind is about midway in your seat.
- Inhale, and as you do, lift your right leg, bend at the knee, and place your right foot on your left thigh.
- Place your right hand on your shin and your left hand on your foot, securing your foot.
- Exhale, and as you do, lean forward slightly by hinging at the hips.
- Hold your pose for 30 seconds.
- Release your pose by placing your right leg on the floor once more.
- Repeat the pose on the other side before returning to your mountain pose.

Modifications

- Easier: Keep your torso upright if leaning forward is too intense.
- Harder: Lean forward more deeply to intensify the stretch.
- Props: Use a cushion under your raised foot if the stretch is too intense.

Tips

- Keep your spine straight, even as you lean forward.
- Avoid forcing your knee down; let it open naturally.

Chair Tree Pose

This pose improves balance and focus.

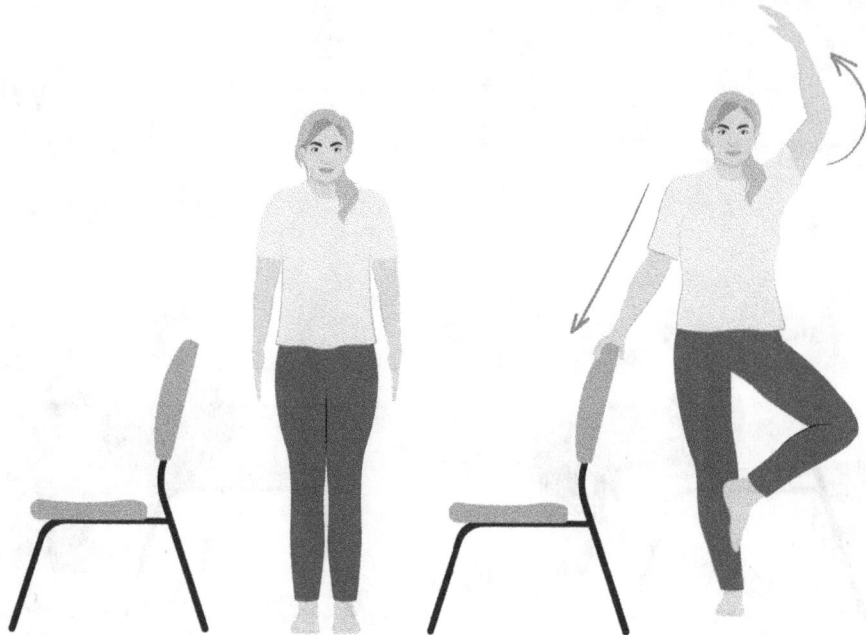

Instructions

- Move your position to the back of your chair and stand with your right side to the backrest.
- Place your right hand on the backrest, inhale, lift your left foot off the floor and engage your core.
- Place the sole of your foot on your calf. Do *not* place your foot on your knee.
- Draw focus to your breath and as you inhale, sweep your left arm up toward the ceiling.
- Keep your elbow slightly bent and your palm facing the ground.
- Gaze forward and hold your pose for 30 seconds.
- Return your left leg to the floor and turn around so your left side faces the backrest.
- Repeat your pose on the other side.

Modifications

- Easier: Keep the raised foot on the ankle instead of the calf.
- Harder: Gaze upward at raised hand.
- Props: Use the chair back for support.

Tips

- Keep your standing leg straight but not locked.
- If you feel unsteady, focus on a fixed point.

Chair Warrior I Pose

This pose strengthens the legs, improves balance, and opens the chest and hips.

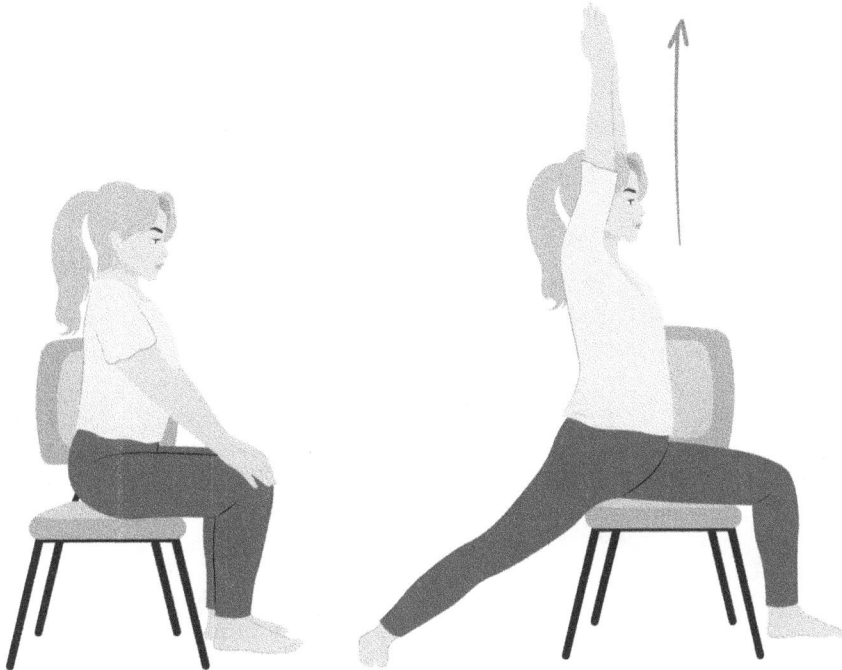

Instructions

- Begin in your neutral mountain pose, feet flat on the floor, and your hands on your thighs.
- Alternatively, begin in a standing position with the seat of your chair between your legs.
- As you inhale, extend your left leg straight behind you. Turn your toes at a slight angle.
- Exhale and turn to the right, bending your right knee with your right foot is planted.
- Inhale and sweep your hands toward the ceiling, palms facing each other.
- Hold your pose for 30 seconds.
- Release by twisting to the front, bending your left knee, and returning to mountain pose.
- Repeat your pose on the other side, extending your right leg behind you.

Modifications

- Easier: Keep hands on the chair seat or armrests for balance.
- Harder: Lift the back heel off the floor for a deeper stretch.
- Props: Use a wall for support if balance is challenging.

Tips

- Keep your front knee aligned over your ankle, not extending past your toes.

Chair Downward Dog

This pose strengthens the upper body, stretches the hamstrings, and promotes better circulation throughout the body.

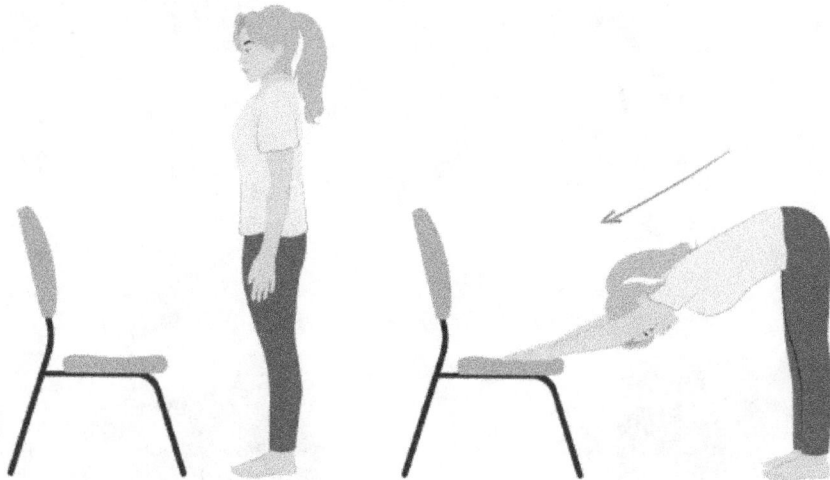

Instructions

- Begin by standing in front of your chair.
- Place your hands on the seating area of your chair.
- On an inhale, take a big step back, allowing your arms to straighten and your head to gaze between your arms.
- As you exhale, straighten your knees and attempt to sink further into your stretch.
- Hold this position for 1 minute.
- To release, slowly roll up to a standing position.
- Take your seat and enter into your mountain pose.

Modifications

- Easier: Keep a slight bend in your knees and focus on lengthening your spine rather than straightening your legs.
- Harder: If flexibility allows, walk your hands further to the back of the seat.
- Props: Place yoga blocks under your hands if you can't reach the seat comfortably.

Tips

- Keep your neck relaxed and in line with your spine.
- Engage your core to protect your lower back.
- Push your hips back into the chair to deepen the stretch in your hamstrings.
- If you feel any sharp pain, especially in your lower back, come out of the pose gently.

Chair Warrior II Pose

This pose strengthens the legs, opens the hips and chest, and improves balance and focus.

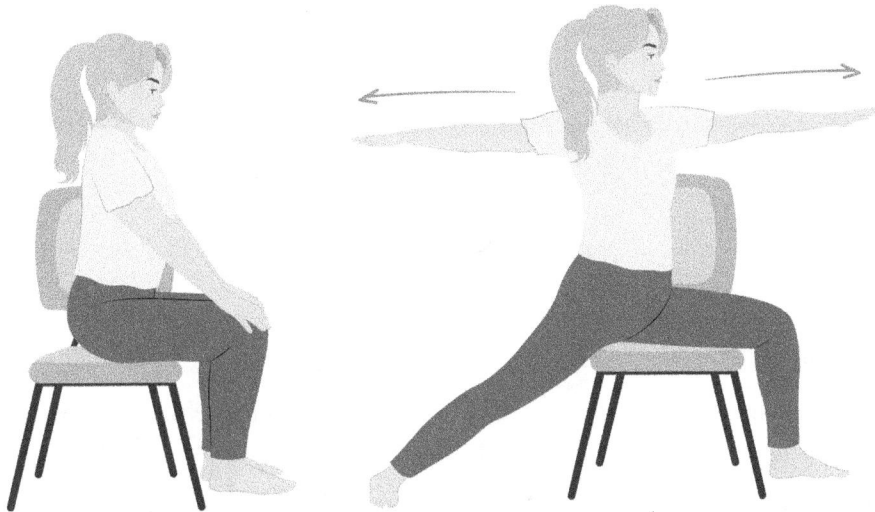

<u>Instructions</u>

- Begin in your neutral mountain pose, feet flat on the floor and hands resting on your thighs. Move forward in your chair slightly.
- Inhale deeply, and as you do, open your left leg out toward the left. Bend your knee slightly, aligning your ankle and hip to form a 90-degree angle.
- Keep your foot relaxed and your toes pointing to the left.
- Exhale, and as you do, extend the right leg in front, twisting your upper body to the right.
- Ensure your right foot is flat and that your toes are pointing forward.
- Inhale and extend your arms to shoulder level, one behind you to the left and one in front of you to the right. Your palms should face the floor, and your elbows should be straight.
- Exhale and turn your gaze to your right. Hold your pose for 30 seconds.
- Release your pose by dropping your arms to your sides and returning both legs to the front of your chair. Place your hands on your thighs and enter the mountain pose again.
- Repeat your pose on the other side.

<u>Modifications</u>

- Easier: Keep hands on the chair seat for balance.
- Harder: Lift the front leg slightly off the floor for an added balance challenge.
- Props: Use blocks under your hands if the floor is too far to reach comfortably.

<u>Tips</u>

- Keep your torso centered between your legs, not leaning forward or back.

Chair Yoga for Weight Loss: Day 8-11

Warm-up: 2 minutes

1. Seated Mountain: 1 minute
2. Seated Forward Bend: 1 minute
3. Seated Spinal Twist: 30 seconds on each side
4. Seated Figure Four: 30 seconds on each side
5. Chair Tree: 1 minute
6. Warrior I: 30 seconds on each side
7. Chair Downward Dog: 1 minute
8. Warrior II: 30 seconds on each side

Tips for Maintaining Proper Form and Alignment

Proper form and alignment are integral to properly engaging your muscles and preventing injuries as you progress to more advanced chair yoga poses.

Alignment begins with your ability to activate your abdominal muscles to support your spine and maintain stability during your chair yoga exercises. Throughout the day, you may unintentionally activate your core, but you need to be able to tap into these stabilizer muscles to maximize your workout consciously. Unfortunately, sedentary lifestyles and office jobs have weakened most people's core muscles, leading to increased lower back pain and telltale weight gain around the lower belly.

The good news is that by properly aligning your spine and consciously correcting your posture, you can begin to activate your core stabilizer muscles once more consciously. Aim to draw your attention to your focus three times a day and consciously lengthen your spine, drop your shoulders back and down, and straighten your pelvis and hips.

Day 12-14: Chair Yoga Poses

Five-Pointed Star

This pose strengthens the legs, opens the chest, and improves overall body awareness.

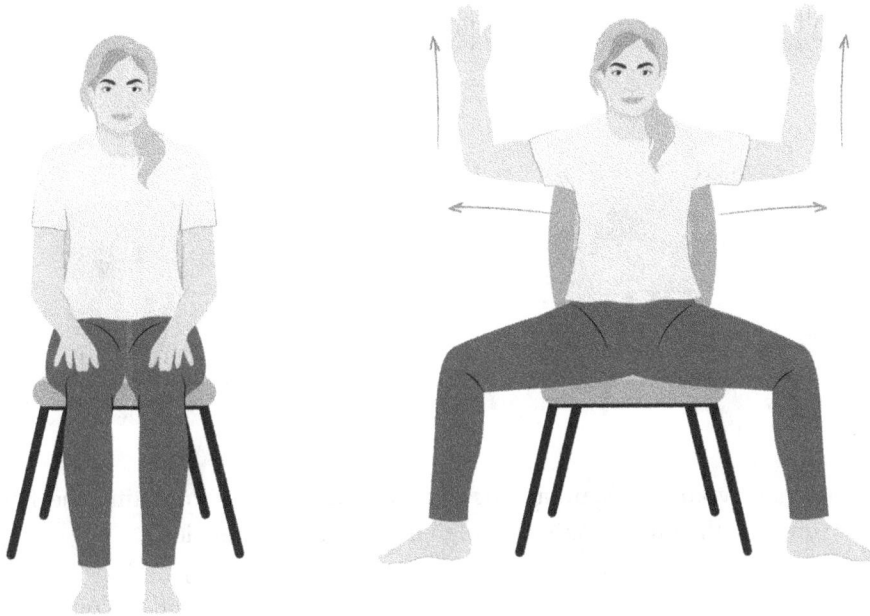

Instructions

- Begin in your neutral mountain pose, feet flat on the floor and your hands on your thighs.
- Inhale and open your legs, widening them to more than hip-width apart.
- Point your toes out at a 45-degree angle and lengthen your spine.
- Exhale and gaze forward.
- Inhale and sweep your arms out to your sides. Keep your elbows straight and your palms facing away from your body.
- Exhale and bend your arms. Spread your fingers wide. Inhale and engage your core.
- Exhale and drop your shoulders back into a relaxed position. Hold your pose for 1 minute.

Modifications

- Easier: Keep arms lower if shoulder mobility is limited.
- Harder: Lift heels off the floor, balancing on toes.
- Props: Use the chair back for support if balance is challenging.

Tips

- Keep your spine straight and chest open throughout the pose.

Seated Spinal Twist

This pose enhances spinal mobility, relieves back tension, and can aid digestion.

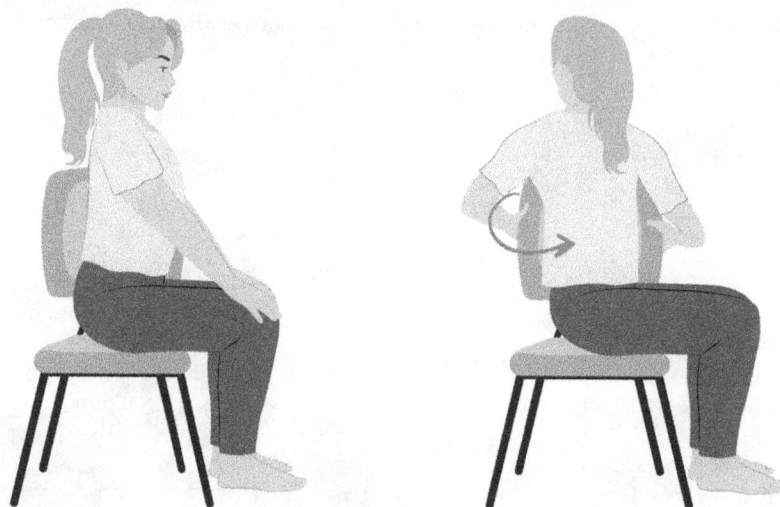

The spinal twist activates your parasympathetic nervous system by stimulating the PSOAS (a pair of large muscles that run from the lumbar spine through the groin on either side).

Instructions

- Turn sideways in your chair, resting your feet flat on the floor.
- Place the hand closest to the backrest on the seating area and your other hand on your thigh.
- Inhale, drop your shoulders back, and turn your gaze to the backrest.
- Exhale and twist your upper torso toward the backrest.
- Place both hands on the backrest and guide your upper body to face the backrest while your hips and feet remain in their starting position.
- Hold your pose for 30 seconds.
- Turn around so your other side is against the backrest, and repeat on the other side.

Modifications

- Easier: Keep one hand on the seat if reaching the backrest is uncomfortable.
- Harder: Deepen the twist by looking over your back shoulder.
- Props: Use a chair with a sturdy backrest for support.

Tips

- Move slowly and mindfully into the twist.
- Keep your hips square to the side of the chair, twisting from your mid-back, not your lower back.

Seated Figure Four Stretch

This pose targets the glutes, hips, and piriformis muscles, improving flexibility and reducing lower body tension.

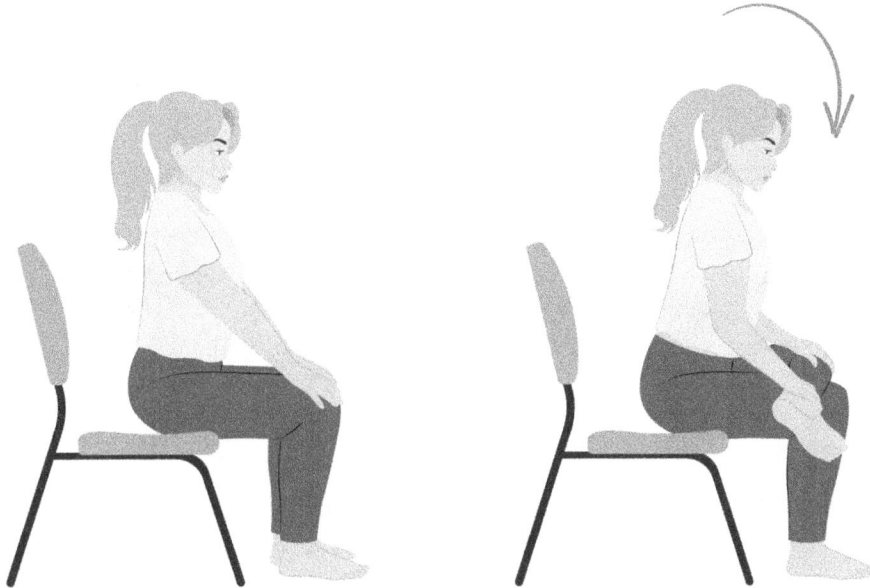

Instructions

- From your mountain pose, sit forward slightly so your behind is about midway in your seat.
- Inhale, and as you do, lift your right leg, bend at the knee, and place your right foot on your left thigh.
- Place your right hand on your shin and your left hand on your foot, securing your foot in place.
- Exhale, and as you do, lean forward slightly by hinging at the hips.
- Hold your pose for 30 seconds.
- Release your pose by placing your right leg on the floor once more.
- Repeat the pose on the other side before returning to your mountain pose.

Modifications

- Easier: Keep your torso upright if leaning forward is too intense.
- Harder: Lean forward more deeply to intensify the stretch.
- Props: Use a cushion under your raised foot if the stretch is too intense.

Tips

- Keep your spine straight, even as you lean forward.
- Avoid forcing your knee down; let it open naturally.

Chair Seated Boat Pose

This pose strengthens the core and improves balance.

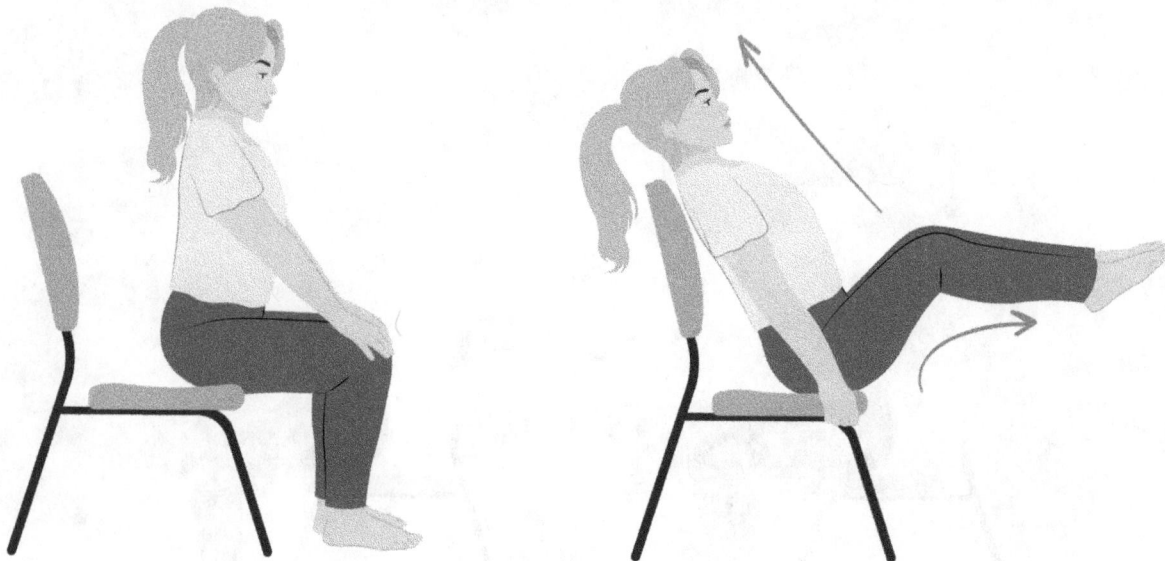

Instructions

- Begin in your neutral mountain pose, feet flat on the floor and your hands resting on your thighs. Shift slightly forward in your chair.
- Inhale deeply, and as you drop your hands to your sides, grip the chair seating and lift your legs up and off the floor.
- Engage your core as you lift your legs, keeping your knees bent.
- Feel free to lean back slightly in your chair, but do not use the backrest for support.
- Hold your pose for 30 seconds.
- Slowly lower your feet to the floor and return your hands to your thighs.

Modifications

- Easier: Keep your feet closer to the floor.
- Harder: Extend legs fully if possible.
- Props: Use a strap around your feet for support.

Tips

- Keep the spine straight throughout the pose.
- Breathe steadily, focusing on core engagement.
- If you feel strain in your lower back, reduce the leg lift.

Chair Warrior I Pose

This pose strengthens the legs, improves balance, and opens the chest and hips.

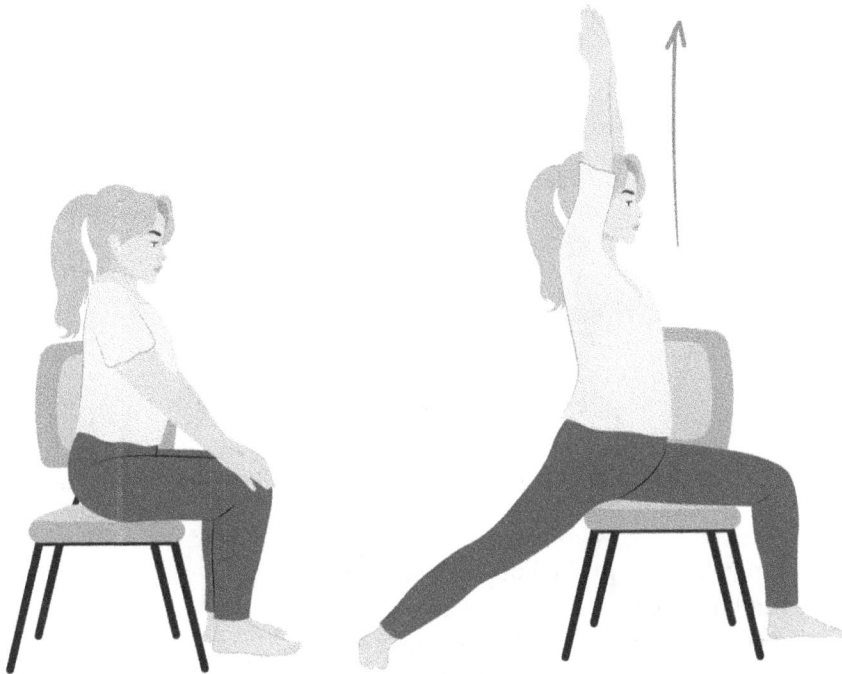

<u>Instructions</u>

- Begin in your neutral mountain pose, feet flat on the floor and your hands on your thighs.
- Alternatively, begin your exercise in a standing position with your chair between your legs.
- As you inhale, extend your left leg straight behind you. Turn your toes at a slight angle.
- Exhale and turn to the right, bending your right knee and ensuring your right foot is planted.
- Inhale and sweep your hands toward the ceiling, palms facing each other.
- Hold your pose for 1 minute.
- Release your pose by twisting your body to the front and bending your left knee.
- Repeat your pose on the other side, extending your right leg behind you.

<u>Modifications</u>

- Easier: Keep hands on the chair seat or armrests for balance.
- Harder: Lift the back heel off the floor for a deeper stretch.
- Props: Use a wall for support if balance is challenging.

<u>Tips</u>

- Keep your front knee aligned over your ankle, not extending past your toes.

Chair Revolved Half Moon Pose

This pose improves balance, strengthens the legs, and stretches the hamstrings and spine.

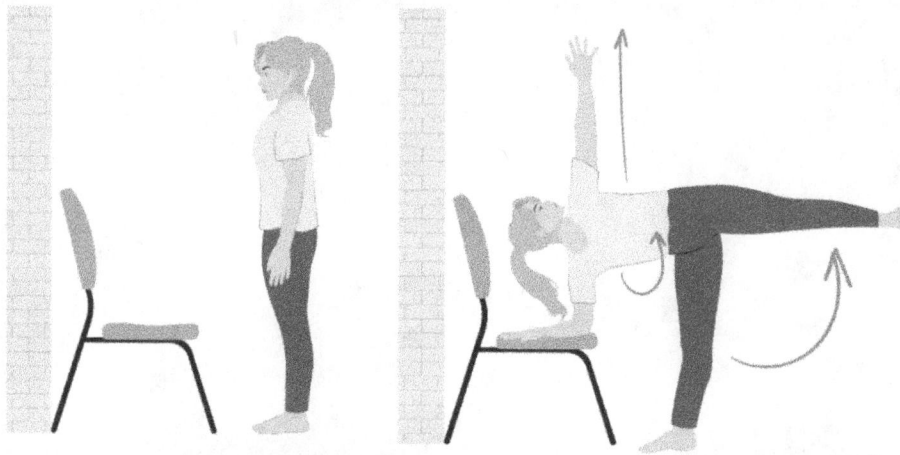

Instructions

- Have the backrest of your chair pushed up against a wall.
- Stand with your right hip facing the seating area of the chair.
- Take a step away from your chair about half an arm's length.
- Inhale, and as you do, drop your right arm to the seating area.
- Exhale and extend your left leg out straight to your side.
- Ensure your right toes are pointing toward the chair and your left foot is in the flexed position.
- Inhale and sweep your left arm up toward the ceiling. Turn your gaze to your left arm.
- Hold your pose for 30 seconds.
- To release from your pose, push up through your arm, place your left foot back on the floor, and enter an upright standing position.
- Turn around so that your left hip is facing the chair.
- Inhale, drop your left arm to the seating area and repeat the pose on the other side.

Modifications

- Easier: Keep the raised leg's toes on the floor for balance.
- Harder: Try to touch the floor instead of the chair seat.
- Props: Chair, wall.

Tips

- Keep the standing leg slightly bent to protect the knee.
- Engage your core for stability.
- If balance is challenging, focus your gaze on a fixed point.

Chair Warrior II Pose

This pose strengthens the legs, opens the hips and chest, and improves balance and focus.

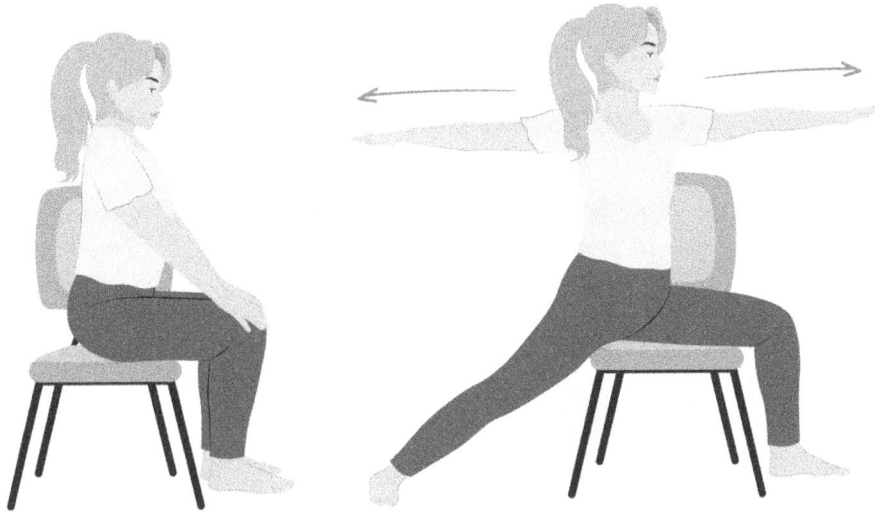

Instructions

- Begin in your neutral mountain pose, feet flat on the floor and hands resting on your thighs. Move forward in your chair slightly.
- Inhale deeply, and as you do, open your left leg out toward the left. Bend your knee slightly, aligning your ankle and hip to form a 90-degree angle.
- Keep your foot relaxed and your toes pointing to the left.
- Exhale, and as you do, extend the right leg in front, twisting your upper body to the right.
- Ensure your right foot is flat and that your toes are pointing forward.
- Inhale and extend your arms to shoulder level, one behind you to the left and one in front of you to the right. Your palms should face the floor, and your elbows should be straight.
- Exhale and turn your gaze to your right. Hold your pose for 30 seconds.
- Release your pose by dropping your arms to your sides and returning both legs to the front.
- Repeat your pose on the other side.

Modifications

- Easier: Keep hands on the chair seat for balance.
- Harder: Lift the front leg slightly off the floor for an added balance challenge.
- Props: Use blocks under your hands if the floor is too far to reach comfortably.

Tips

- Keep your torso centered between your legs, not leaning forward or back.
- Engage your core for stability.

Chair Camel Pose

This pose opens the chest, stretches the front body, and strengthens the back muscles.

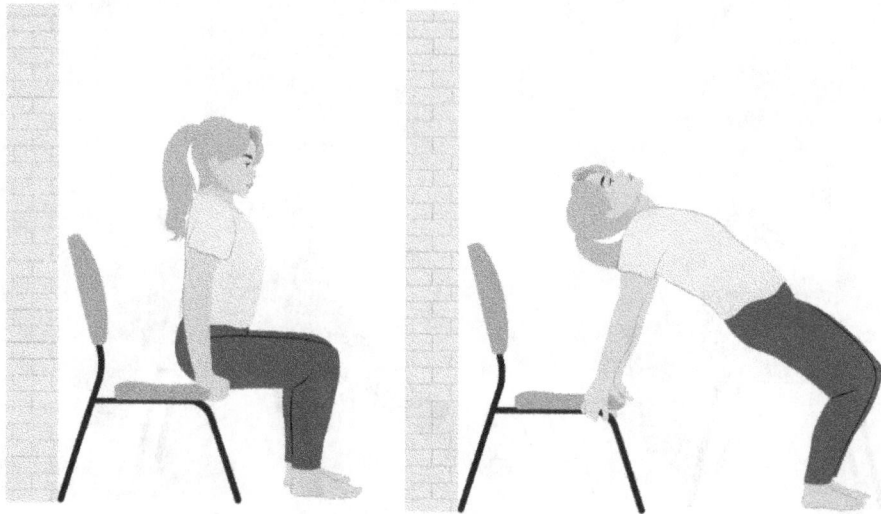

Instructions

- Have the backrest of your chair pushed up against a wall.
- Begin in your neutral mountain pose, feet flat on the floor, and your hands resting on your thighs.
- Inhale and drop your hands to your sides, grasping hold of the seating area of your chair.
- Exhale and open your legs about hip-width apart.
- Inhale and press up with your arms.
- Keep your knees slightly bent and your toes facing forward.
- Exhale and gaze up at the ceiling.
- Hold your pose for 1 minute.
- Return to your chair by walking your feet back, bending your elbows, and carefully sitting down.
- Stand up from your chair and come to the floor in front of your chair facing your seating area.

Modifications

- Easier: Keep hips on the chair seat; just arch the upper back.
- Harder: Try to lift hips higher for a deeper backbend.
- Props: Chair, wall.

Tips

- Warm up back thoroughly before this pose.
- Keep your neck in line with your spine; don't drop your head back.

Chair Yoga for Weight Loss: Day 12 to 14

Warm-up: 2 minutes

1. Seated Five-Pointed Star: 1 minute
2. Seated Spinal Twist: 30 seconds on each side
3. Seated Figure Four: 30 seconds on each side
4. Seated Boat: 1 minute
5. Warrior I: 30 seconds on each side
6. Revolved Half-Moon: 30 seconds on each side
7. Warrior II: 30 seconds on each side
8. Seated Camel: 1 minute

Vinyasa for the Core

Another fantastic way to begin engaging your core muscles is to practice vinyasa. This is a sequence of poses linked together in a fluid, flowing movement. If you're unsure how to correct your posture or simply cannot step away from your desk during the day, vinyasa can be used for a quick core-boosting workout.

- Begin in your mountain pose with your feet flat on the floor and your hands resting on your thighs.
- Inhale and lift your right foot off the floor.
- Place your right sole on your left thigh and press your right knee towards the floor.
- Hold as you exhale and inhale.
- Exhale and release your right foot back to the floor.
- Inhale and lift your arms over your head, reaching your fingertips to the ceiling, palms facing each other.
- Hold, and you exhale and inhale once more.
- Exhale, hinge at the hips, and sweep your arms down to the floor, flattening your upper body to your thighs.
- Hold as you inhale and exhale.
- Inhale and sit upright, placing your hands on your thighs.
- Hold as you exhale, inhale, and exhale once more.
- Inhale and lift your left foot off the floor, pressing the sole of your foot into your right thigh.
- Complete the entire sequence again.

This first vinyasa will integrate you slowly into conscious alignment and core engagement and can be extended as your body becomes stronger. While vinyasa is not particularly challenging, it's important not to dive right in and flow between all of your chair yoga exercises.

Instead, allow your body to progress at its own pace.

CHAPTER 6
WEEK 3—DEEPENING YOUR PRACTICE

*T*his week, you will begin to take on more advanced chair yoga poses. These poses will test your strength and endurance, so it's vital that you remain within your limits and use props and modifications should a pose feel uncomfortable.

This week, you will focus on strengthening your core for your final week of chair yoga. Proper alignment and stability are critical for a strong core. I encourage you to take your poses seriously. Instead, focus on your breath and how your body feels as you engage and move through each pose.

Intermediate Chair Yoga Poses

While some poses may be more challenging, most will still be achievable. Take time, breathe through each stretch, and celebrate your body as it strengthens.

For some of these exercises, you will need a second chair or chair placed next to a steady piece of furniture. You may also require yoga blocks and straps or substitutes.

Day 15-18: Chair Yoga Poses

Seated Mountain Pose

This foundational pose promotes proper alignment, improves posture, and centers the body and mind.

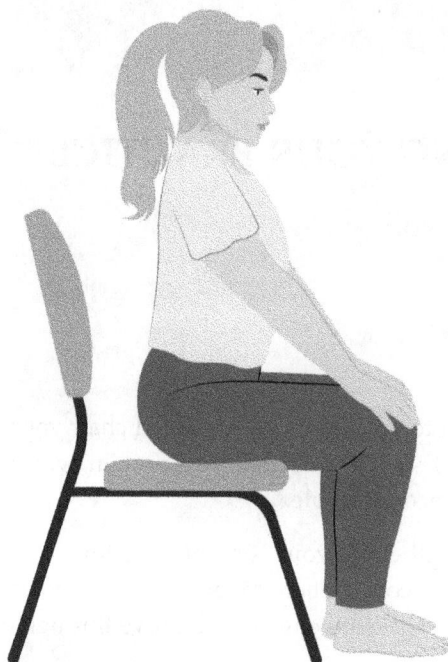

Instructions

- Sit tall in your chair with your feet in front of you, and feet flat on the floor.
- Rest your hands on your knees, palms down, and gaze forward in a neutral position.
- Inhale deeply, and as you exhale, press down into your sitting bones and lengthen your spine.
- As you inhale, engage your core, roll your shoulders back and down, and lift your chest.
- Remain in your mountain pose for 1 minute.

Modifications

- Easier: Use a chair with back support if needed.
- Harder: Close your eyes to increase body awareness.
- Props: Place a folded blanket under your feet if they don't reach the floor.

Tips

- Relax your face and jaw while maintaining the posture.

Seated Wide-Legged Forward Fold

This pose stretches the inner thighs, hamstrings, and lower back.

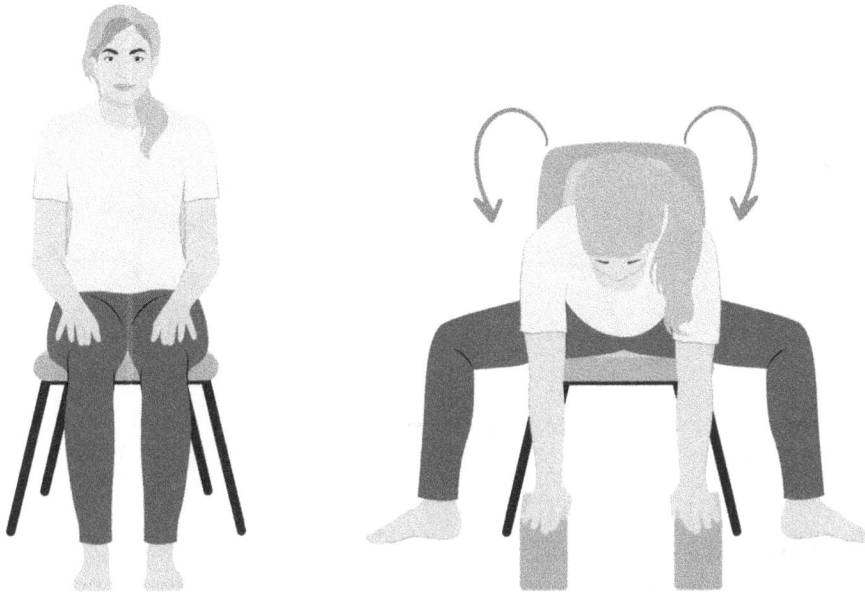

Instructions

- Begin in your neutral mountain pose, feet flat on the floor and your hands on your thighs.
- Inhale and sweep your arms toward the ceiling, palms facing each other.
- Exhale and open your legs to slightly wider than hip-width apart.
- Inhale deeply, lengthening your spine and reaching up further toward the ceiling.
- Exhale and sweep your arms forward, hinging at the hips.
- Control your movements as you reach for the floor.
- Use yoga blocks or books to bring the floor closer to your hands.
- Keep your gaze aligned with your spine and your feet firmly planted on the floor.
- Hold your pose for 1 minute.
- To return to your center, inhale and lift your torso to a seated position.

Modifications

- Easier: Bend knees slightly if hamstrings are tight.
- Harder: Grasp the outer edges of feet if flexibility allows.
- Props: Use yoga blocks or books to "raise" the floor.

Tips

- Keep your back straight as you fold forward.

Seated Half Lotus Pose

This pose improves hip flexibility and promotes inner calm.

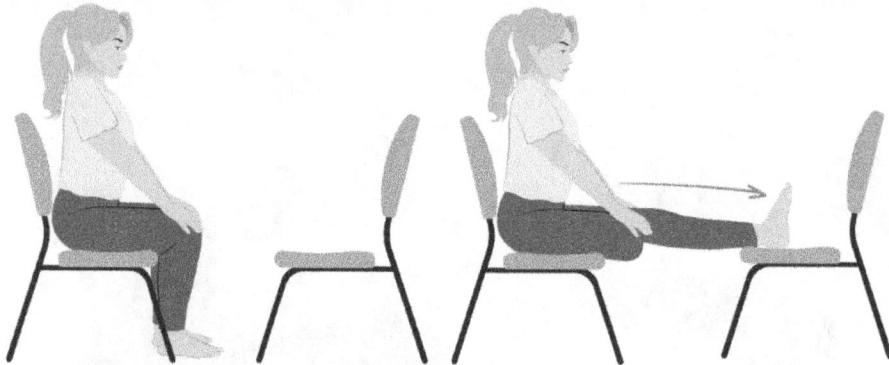

You will need an extra chair or sturdy piece of furniture for this pose.

<u>Instructions</u>

- Turn your chair so that the seating areas face each other.
- Leave about a chair's width between each chair.
- Begin in neutral mountain pose, feet on the floor and your hands resting on your thighs.
- Inhale and bend. Lift your right leg, bend it at the knee, and place the sole of your foot on your left thigh.
- Exhale and move your hands to your hips, gazing straight ahead.
- Inhale once more and lift your left leg off the floor, straightening it and bringing your heel to rest on the chair in front of you.
- Exhale and lengthen your spine.
- Inhale again, engage your core, and lift your left leg slightly.
- Press your right foot into your left thigh for extra stability, and hold your pose for 30 seconds.
- Release your pose as you exhale, bringing your left and right legs to the floor.
- Place your hands on your thighs to enter a mountain pose before completing your pose on the other side.

<u>Modifications</u>

- Easier: Keep the bottom foot on the floor if lifting is too challenging.
- Harder: Try to straighten the extended leg more.
- Props: Two chairs or a sturdy piece of furniture.

<u>Tips</u>

- Don't force your foot onto the opposite thigh if it's uncomfortable.
- Keep your spine straight throughout the pose.

Chair High Lunge

This pose strengthens legs and improves balance.

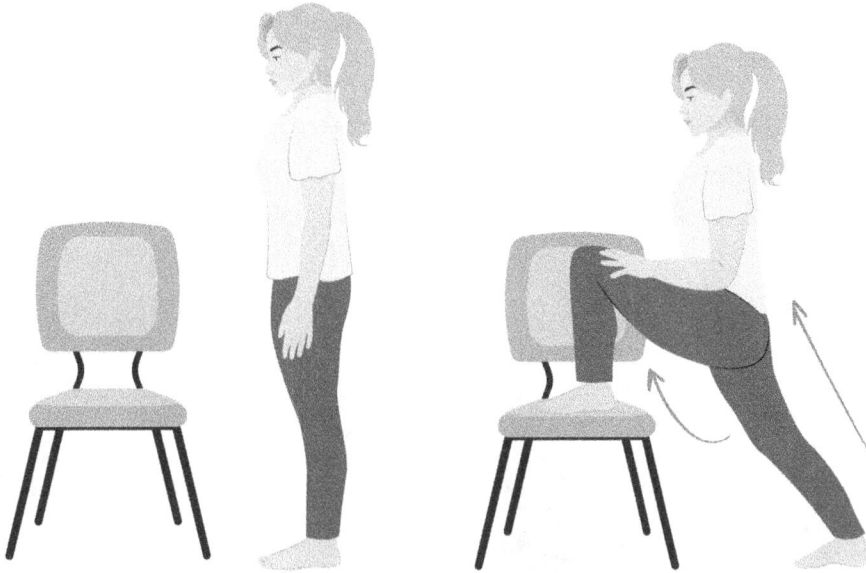

<u>Instructions</u>

- Stand up and face your chair's seating area.
- Step back so you're about half a leg's length from the chair.
- Inhale, lift your right foot off the floor, and place the sole on the seat of the chair.
- Bring attention to your breath and your balance. If you need more balance, realign your left foot.
- On your next inhale, place your hands on your right thigh and lean forward, bending your right knee more and straightening your back leg.
- Hold the pose for 30 seconds.
- Release your pose by stepping down with your right leg.
- Inhale and lift your left leg, bending your knee and placing your foot on the chair.
- Repeat your pose on the other side.

<u>Modifications</u>

- Easier: Keep your back knee bent slightly or hold on to the back of the chair for support.
- Harder: Raise arms overhead.
- Props: Use the chair back for balance if needed.

<u>Tips</u>

- Keep the front knee aligned over the ankle.
- Engage the core for stability and breathe steadily, focusing on balance.

Chair Tree Pose

This pose improves balance and focus.

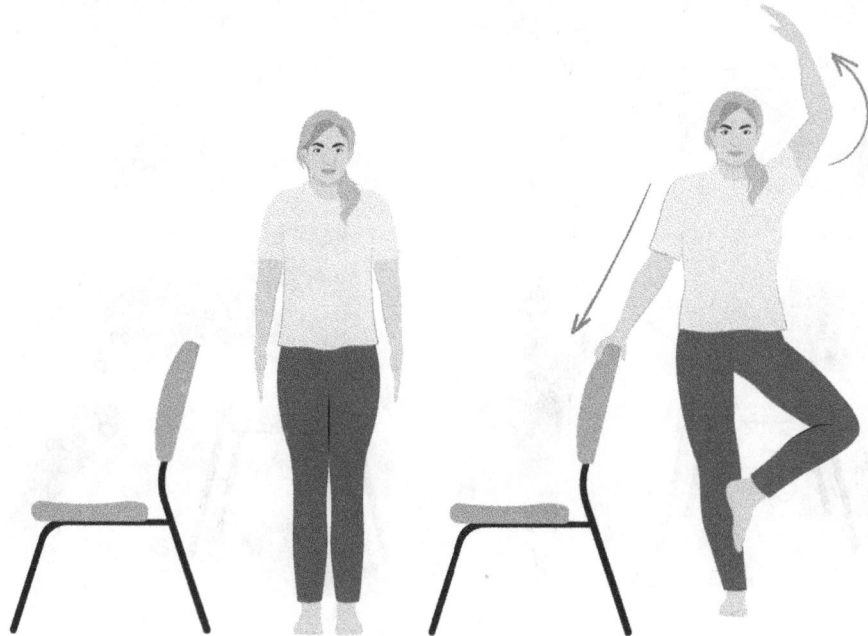

Instructions

- Move your position to the back of your chair and stand with your right side to the backrest.
- Place your right hand on the backrest, inhale, lift your left foot off the floor and engage your core.
- Place the sole of your foot on your calf. Do *not* place your foot on your knee.
- Draw focus to your breath and as you inhale, sweep your left arm up toward the ceiling.
- Keep your elbow slightly bent and your palm facing the ground.
- Gaze forward and hold your pose for 30 seconds.
- Return your left leg to the floor and turn around so your left side faces the backrest.
- Repeat your pose on the other side.

Modifications

- Easier: Keep the raised foot on the ankle instead of the calf.
- Harder: Gaze upward at raised hand.
- Props: Use the chair back for support.

Tips

- Keep your standing leg straight but not locked.
- Engage the core for stability.

Chair Revolved Triangle Pose

This pose improves balance, stretches the hamstrings, and twists the spine.

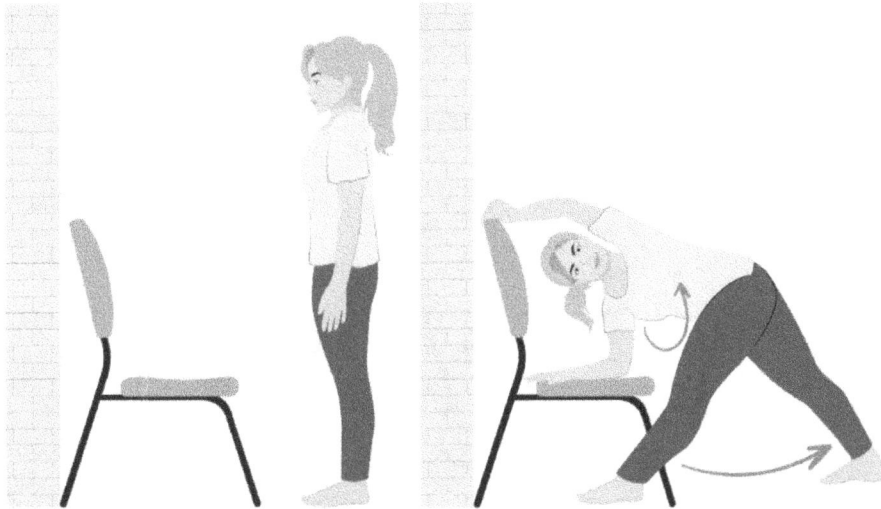

Instructions

- Have the backrest of your chair pushed up against a wall and stand facing your chair's seat.
- Take a step away from your chair about a full body length.
- Have both feet facing toward your chair and your legs about hip-width apart.
- Inhale, and as you do, take a big step forward with your right foot.
- Aim to have the toes of your right foot about a quarter of the way under your chair.
- Exhale, straighten your legs, hinge at your hips, lowering your left forearm to your chair.
- Inhale, place your right arm on the backrest of your chair, and twist your body to the right.
- Gaze over to your right and hold your pose for 30 seconds.
- Inhale, step your left leg forward, hinge at your hips, and return to an upright position.
- On your next exhale, take a big step back, and repeat your pose on the other side.
- Return to your neutral standing position and turn your back to your chair.

Modifications

- Easier: Bend the front knee slightly if the hamstrings are tight.
- Harder: Reach the bottom hand to the floor instead of the chair seat.
- Props: Chair, wall.

Tips

- Keep both legs straight but not locked.
- Twist from your mid-back, not your lower back.
- If balance is challenging, focus your gaze on a fixed point.

Chair Revolved Half Moon Pose

This pose improves balance, strengthens the legs, and stretches the hamstrings and spine.

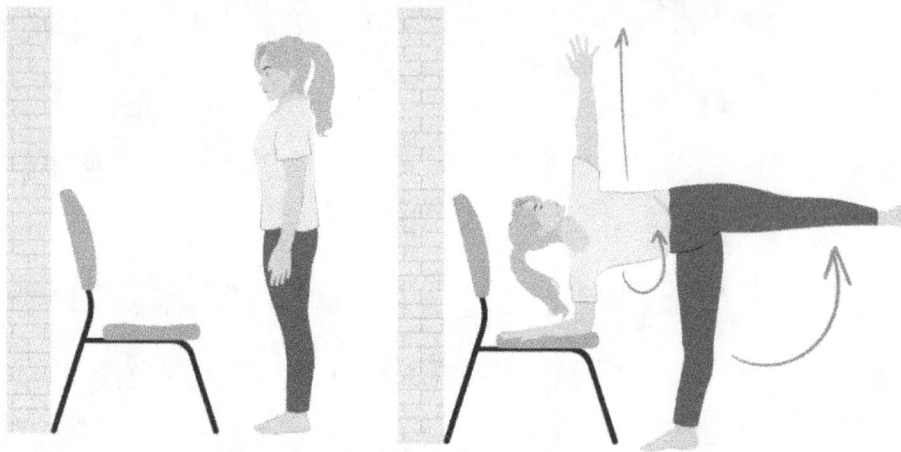

Instructions

- Have the backrest of your chair pushed up against a wall.
- Stand with your right hip facing the seating area of the chair.
- Take a step away from your chair about half an arm's length.
- Inhale, and as you do, drop your right arm to the seating area.
- Exhale and extend your left leg out straight to your side.
- Ensure your right toes are pointing toward the chair and your left foot is in the flexed position.
- Inhale and sweep your left arm up toward the ceiling. Turn your gaze to your left arm.
- Hold your pose for 30 seconds.
- To release from your pose, push up through your arm, place your left foot back on the floor, and enter an upright standing position.
- Turn around so that your left hip is facing the chair.
- Inhale, drop your left arm to the seating area and repeat the pose on the other side.

Modifications

- Easier: Keep the raised leg's toes on the floor for balance.
- Harder: Try to touch the floor instead of the chair seat.
- Props: Chair, wall.

Tips

- Keep the standing leg slightly bent to protect the knee.
- Engage your core for stability.
- If balance is challenging, focus your gaze on a fixed point.

Chair Cobra

This pose strengthens the back muscles, improves posture, and helps counteract the effects of prolonged sitting by opening the chest and shoulders.

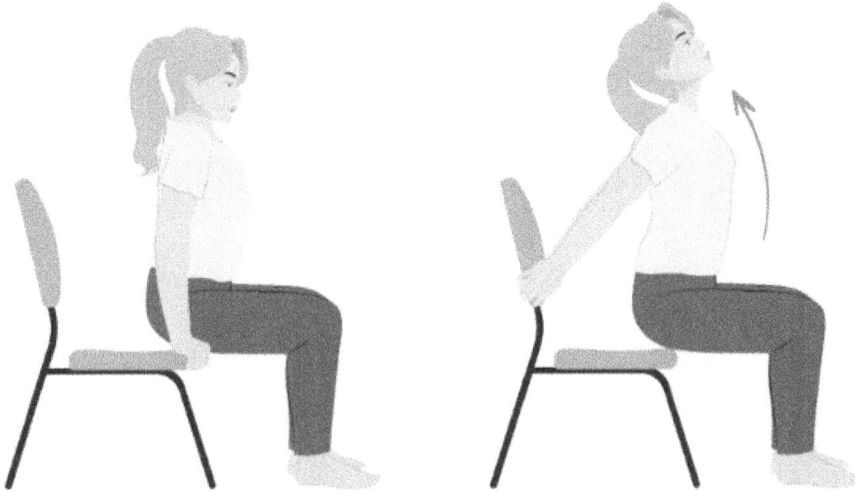

<u>Instructions</u>

- Sit towards the front edge of a sturdy chair with your feet flat on the floor, hip-width apart.
- Place your hands on your thighs, palms down.
- On an inhale, slide your hands back towards your hips, gripping the backrest of your chair.
- As you exhale, lift your chest, arching your back slightly.
- Roll your shoulders back and down, away from your ears.
- Lift your chin slightly, gazing forward or slightly upward.
- Keep your buttocks and legs engaged, pressing into the chair and floor.
- Hold this position for 1 minute.
- To release, slowly lower your chest and return to a neutral seated position on an exhale.

<u>Modifications</u>

- Easier: Perform a gentler bend, focusing on opening the chest rather than arching the back.
- Harder: If flexibility allows, lift your buttocks slightly off the chair, intensifying the backbend.
- Props: Use a small cushion for lower back support if needed.

<u>Tips</u>

- Keep your neck in line with your spine, avoiding excessive backward tilting of the head.
- Engage your core muscles to protect your lower back and focus on lifting through the sternum rather than compressing the lower back.
- If you feel any pinching in your lower back, reduce the intensity of the backbend.

Chair Yoga for Weight Loss: Day 15 to 18

Warm-up: 2 minutes

1. Seated Mountain: 1 minute
2. Wide-Legged Forward Fold: 1 minute
3. Seated Half Lotus: 30 seconds on each side
4. High Lunge: 30 seconds on each side
5. Chair Tree: 30 seconds on each side
6. Chair Revolved Triangle: 30 seconds on each side
7. Chair Revolved Half Moon: 30 seconds on each side
8. Chair Cobra: 1 minute

Alternatives to Traditional Yoga Props

Yoga props can enhance your practice, but you don't need specialized equipment to get started with chair yoga. Many common household items can serve as excellent alternatives.

- A sturdy hardcover book can replace a yoga block, providing support in forward bends or seated poses.
- Cushions or folded blankets can offer extra height or padding, making seated poses more comfortable.
- A bath towel or scarf can substitute for a yoga strap, helping you reach your feet in stretches like Seated Extended Hand-to-Big-Toe Pose.
- Resistance bands are great alternatives to yoga straps for deepening stretches or assisting in poses requiring more flexibility.
- Rolled-up magazines can serve as a small bolster to support your lower back or knees.

Remember, the goal is to make your practice accessible and comfortable, so feel free to get creative with items you already have at home. The most important thing is to ensure whatever you use is stable and safe for your practice.

Day 19-21: Chair Yoga Poses

Five-Pointed Star

This pose strengthens the legs, opens the chest, and improves overall body awareness.

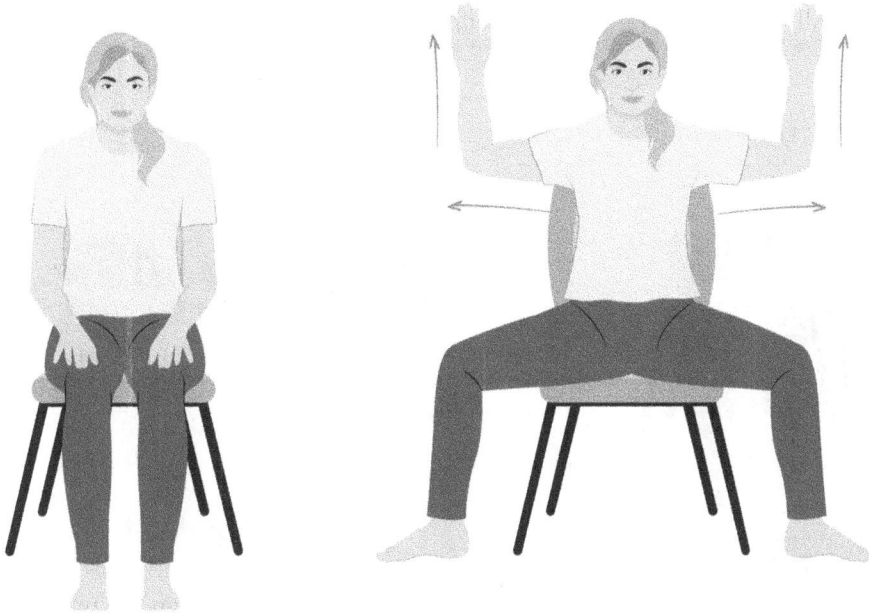

Instructions

- Begin in your neutral mountain pose, feet flat on the floor and your hands on your thighs.
- Inhale and open your legs, widening them to more than hip-width apart.
- Point your toes out at a 45-degree angle and lengthen your spine.
- Exhale and gaze forward.
- Inhale and sweep your arms out to your sides. Keep your elbows straight and your palms facing away from your body.
- Exhale and bend your arms. Spread your fingers wide. Inhale and engage your core.
- Exhale and drop your shoulders back into a relaxed position. Hold your pose for 1 minute.

Modifications

- Easier: Keep arms lower if shoulder mobility is limited.
- Harder: Lift heels off the floor, balancing on toes.
- Props: Use the chair back for support if balance is challenging.

Tips

- Keep your spine straight and chest open throughout the pose.

Seated Wide-Legged Forward Fold

This pose stretches the inner thighs, hamstrings, and lower back.

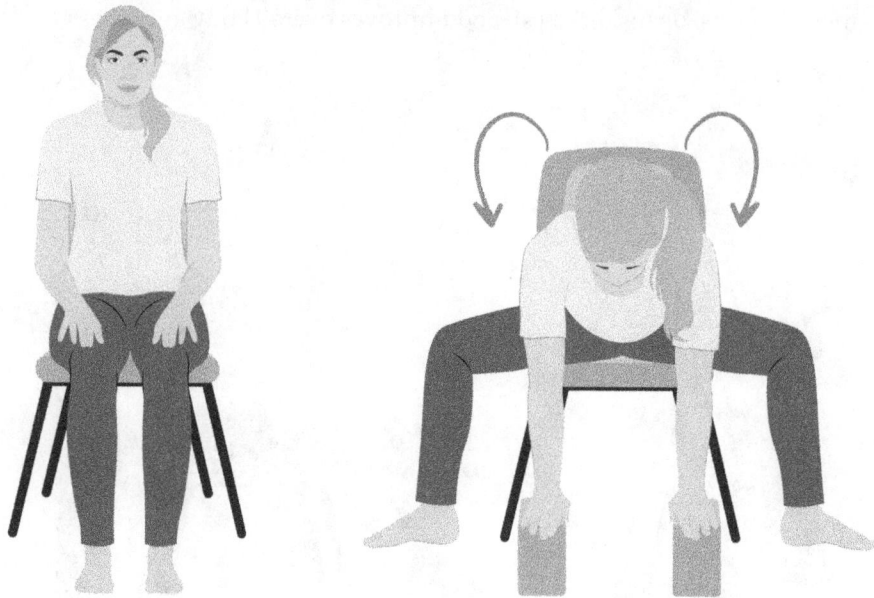

Instructions

- Begin in your neutral mountain pose, feet flat on the floor and your hands on your thighs.
- Inhale and sweep your arms toward the ceiling, palms facing each other.
- Exhale and open your legs to slightly wider than hip-width apart.
- Inhale deeply, lengthening your spine and reaching up further toward the ceiling.
- Exhale and sweep your arms forward, hinging at the hips as you reach for the floor.
- Use yoga blocks or books to bring the floor closer to your hands.
- Keep your gaze aligned with your spine and your feet firmly planted on the floor.
- Hold your pose for 1 minute.
- To return to your center, inhale and lift your torso to a seated position.

Modifications

- Easier: Bend knees slightly if hamstrings are tight.
- Harder: Grasp the outer edges of feet if flexibility allows.
- Props: Use yoga blocks or books to "raise" the floor.

Tips

- Keep your back straight as you fold forward.
- Don't force the stretch; go only as far as comfortable.

Seated Cow Face Pose

This pose stretches the shoulders and upper back. This pose may require a strap, towel, or blanket.

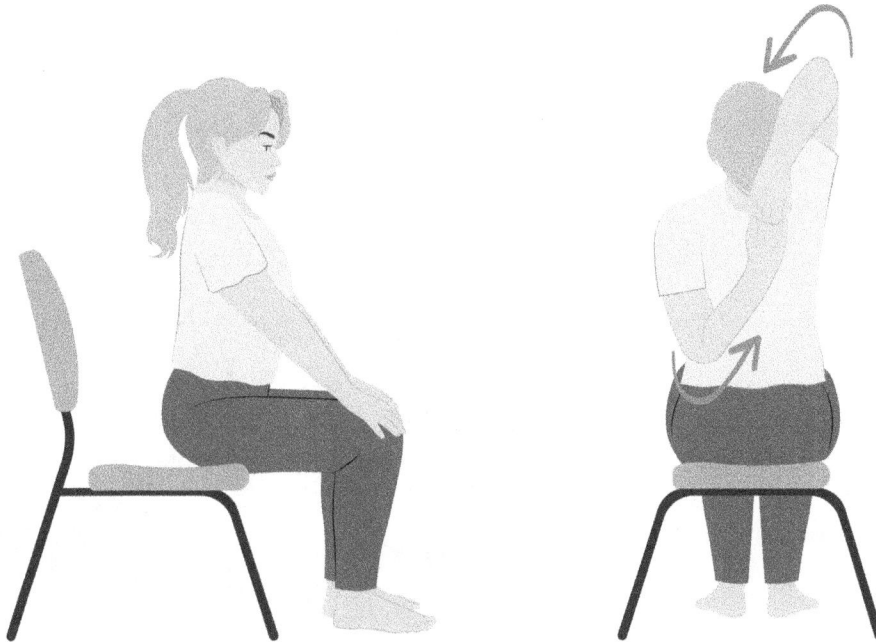

Instructions

- Begin in your neutral mountain pose, feet flat on the floor and your hands resting on your thighs.
- Shift slightly forward, inhale and lengthen your spine. Exhale and plant your feet on the floor.
- On your next inhale, sweep your right arm up toward the ceiling.
- Exhale and sweep your left arm behind you, bending your elbow and reaching up toward your shoulder blades.
- Inhale once more and bend your right arm behind your head and neck. Try to reach your hands to each other or use a strap to connect the space between your hands.
- Hold your pose for 30 seconds.
- Inhale and repeat the pose on the other side before returning to the mountain pose.

Modifications

- Easier: Keep the bottom elbow lower if the shoulders are tight.
- Harder: Pull on the strap to deepen the stretch.
- Props: Hold a yoga strap, towel, or blanket between your hands if you cannot reach.

Tips

- Keep your spine straight and your shoulders relaxed.

Chair Upward Plank Pose

This pose strengthens arms, shoulders, and core while opening the chest.

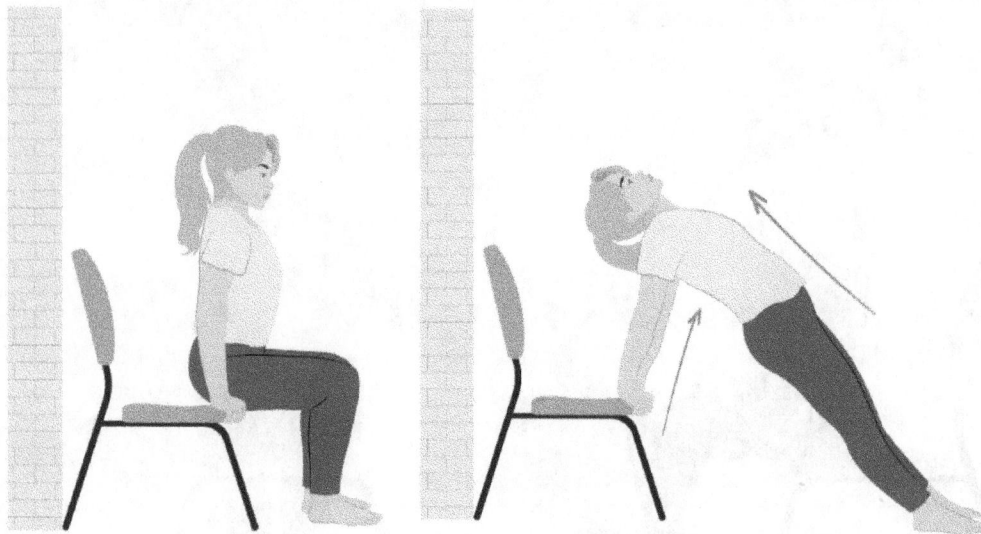

Instructions

- Have the backrest of your chair pushed up against a wall.
- Sit on the very edge of your chair, place your hands on the front edge, and grip your chair tightly.
- Straighten your legs out straight in front of you.
- Inhale, and as you do, push up through your arms, lifting your body off the chair in a straight line.
- Engage your core and straighten your neck, gazing upward toward the ceiling.
- Hold your pose for 1 minute.
- To release your pose, take a step back, slowly bend your elbows, and place your buttocks on the seat.

Modifications

- Easier: Keep knees bent.
- Harder: Lift one leg at a time off the floor.
- Props: Chair, wall.

Tips

- Keep shoulders away from ears.
- Engage glutes and leg muscles.
- If wrists hurt, make fists or use yoga blocks on the chair.

Chair Warrior I Pose

This pose strengthens the legs, improves balance, and opens the chest and hips.

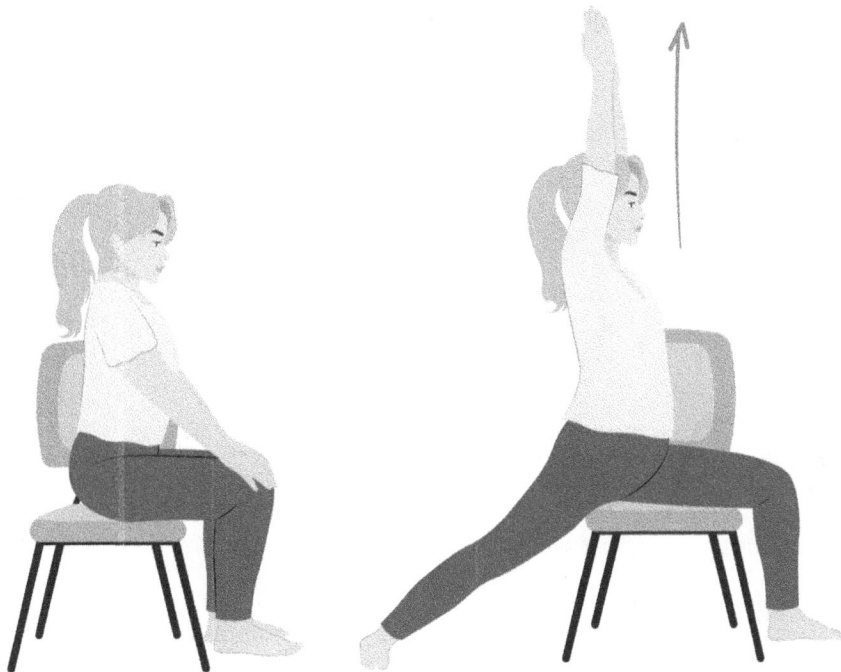

Instructions

- Begin in your neutral mountain pose, feet flat on the floor and your hands on your thighs.
- Alternatively, begin your exercise in a standing position with your chair between your legs.
- Inhale, extend your left leg straight behind you. Turn your toes at a 45-degree angle.
- Exhale and turn to the right, bending your right knee and ensuring your foot is planted.
- Inhale and sweep your hands toward the ceiling, palms facing each other.
- Hold your pose for 1 minute.
- Release your pose by twisting your body to the front and bending your left knee.
- Repeat your pose on the other side, extending your right leg behind you.

Modifications

- Easier: Keep hands on the chair seat or armrests for balance.
- Harder: Lift the back heel off the floor for a deeper stretch.
- Props: Use a wall for support if balance is challenging.

Tips

- Keep your front knee aligned over your ankle, not extending past your toes.

Chair Downward Dog

This pose strengthens the upper body, stretches the hamstrings, and promotes better circulation throughout the body.

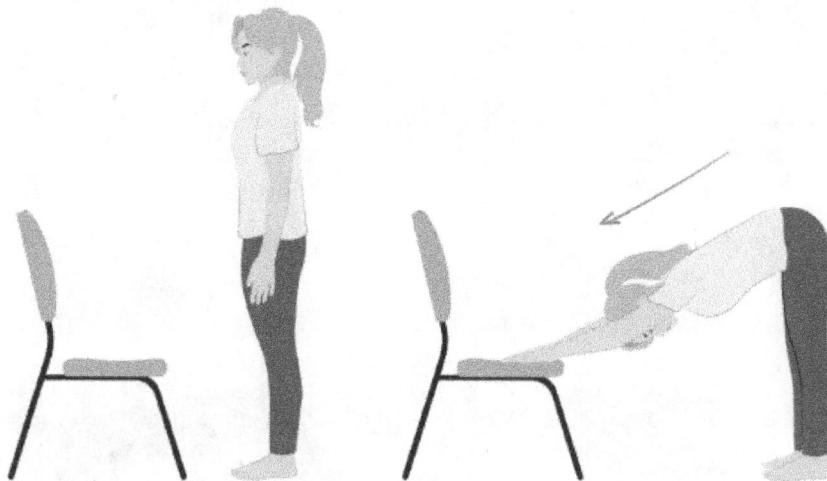

Instructions

- Begin by standing in front of your chair.
- Place your hands on the seating area of your chair.
- On an inhale, take a big step back, allowing your arms to straighten and your head to gaze between your arms.
- As you exhale, straighten your knees and attempt to sink further into your stretch.
- Hold this position for 1 minute.
- To release, slowly roll up to a standing position.

Modifications

- Easier: Keep a slight bend in your knees and focus on lengthening your spine rather than straightening your legs.
- Harder: If flexibility allows, walk your hands further forward the back of your seat, intensifying the stretch.
- Props: Place yoga blocks under your hands if you can't reach the seat comfortably.

Tips

- Keep your neck relaxed and in line with your spine.
- Engage your core to protect your lower back, pushing your hips back into the chair to deepen the stretch in your hamstrings.
- Breathe deeply and evenly throughout the pose.

Chair Warrior II Pose

This pose strengthens the legs, opens the hips and chest, and improves balance and focus.

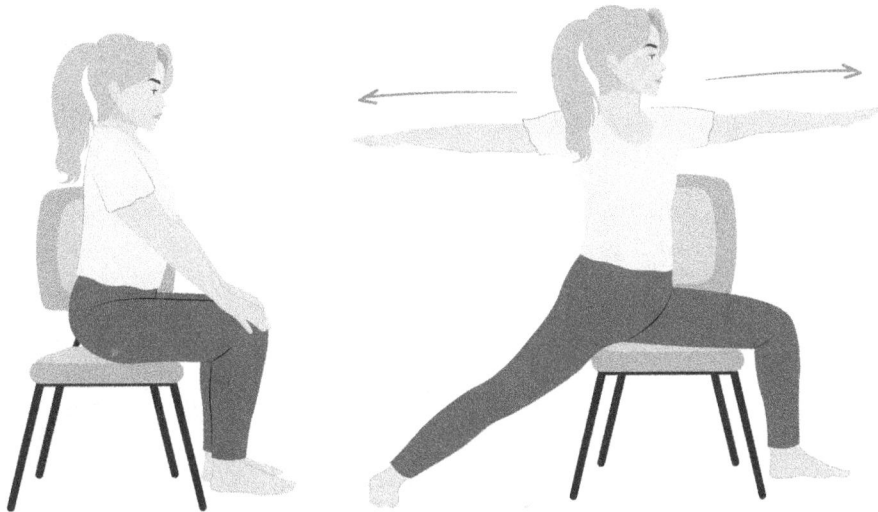

Instructions

- Begin in your neutral mountain pose, feet flat on the floor and hands resting on your thighs. Move forward in your chair slightly.
- Inhale deeply, and as you do, open your left leg out toward the left. Bend your knee slightly, aligning your ankle and hip to form a 90-degree angle.
- Keep your foot relaxed and your toes pointing to the left.
- Exhale, and as you do, extend the right leg in front, twisting your upper body to the right.
- Ensure your right foot is flat and that your toes are pointing forward.
- Inhale and extend your arms to shoulder level, one behind you to the left and one in front of you to the right. Your palms should face the floor, and your elbows should be straight.
- Exhale and turn your gaze to your right. Hold your pose for 30 seconds.
- Release your pose by dropping your arms to your sides and returning both legs to the front of your chair. Place your hands on your thighs and enter the mountain pose again.
- Repeat your pose on the other side.

Modifications

- Easier: Keep hands on the chair seat for balance.
- Harder: Lift the front leg slightly off the floor for an added balance challenge.
- Props: Use blocks under your hands if the floor is too far to reach comfortably.

Tips

- Keep your torso centered between your legs, not leaning forward or back.

Chair Revolved Triangle Pose

This pose improves balance, stretches the hamstrings, and twists the spine.

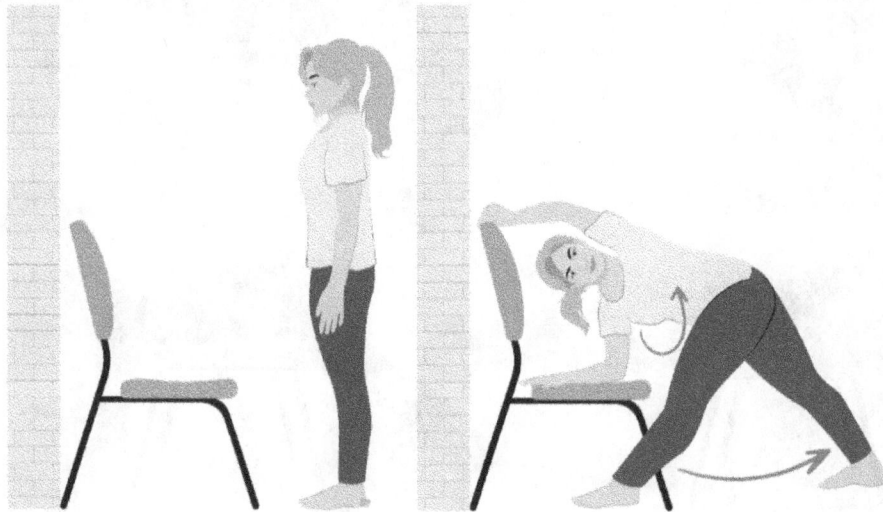

Instructions

- Have the backrest of your chair pushed up against a wall.
- Stand facing your chair's seating area and take a step away from your chair about a full body length.
- Have both feet facing toward your chair and your legs about hip-width apart.
- Inhale, and as you do, take a big step forward with your right foot.
- Aim to have the toes of your right foot about a quarter of the way under your chair's seating area.
- Exhale, straighten your legs, and hinge at your hips, lowering your left forearm to your seating area.
- Inhale, place your right arm on the backrest of your chair, and twist your body to the right.
- Gaze over to your right and hold your pose for 30 seconds.
- Inhale, step your left leg forward, hinge at your hips, and return to an upright position.
- On your next exhale, take a big step back, and repeat your pose on the other side.

Modifications

- Easier: Bend the front knee slightly if the hamstrings are tight.
- Harder: Reach the bottom hand to the floor instead of the chair seat.
- Props: Chair, wall.

Tips

- Keep both legs straight but not locked.
- Twist from your mid-back, not your lower back.

Chair Yoga for Weight Loss: Day 19 to 21

Warm-up: 2 minutes

1. Seated Five-Pointed Star: 1 minute
2. Wide-Legged Forward Fold: 1 minute
3. Seated Cow Face: 30 seconds on each side
4. Upward Plank 1 minute
5. Warrior I: 30 seconds on each side
6. Chair Downward Dog: 1 minute
7. Warrior II: 30 seconds on each side
8. Revolved Triangle: 30 seconds on each side

Now that we have completed Week 3, let's start the last week, where we will explore the most advanced chair yoga poses.

CHAPTER 7
WEEK 4—MASTERING CHAIR YOGA

*A*s you enter the last week of your chair yoga workouts, your poses become more advanced. During this final week, it becomes critical for you to listen to your body and make use of the modifications provided should a pose feel too taxing.

In addition, the poses below further solidify your teachings from previous weeks using elements such as alignment, breathwork, flow (vinyasa), and core engagement. This week, I encourage you to move your chair closer to a wall for more stability and resistance. Having your chair backed against a wall allows you to explore your flexibility and strength without the fear of falling.

Furthermore, I suggest using props to help you complete each pose. This will provide you with a solid foundation to boost your chances of weight loss and tap into your brain's reward system for sustained motivation.

Advanced Poses for Strength and Weight Loss

For this section, please move your chair to a wall and ensure it is on a non-slip, firm grip surface. You will require yoga blocks (or alternatives) and a yoga strap (or alternative). Feel free to use the modifications provided and celebrate each pose that you successfully flow through.

Day 22-25: Chair Yoga Poses

Seated Mountain Pose

This foundational pose promotes proper alignment, improves posture, and centers the body and mind.

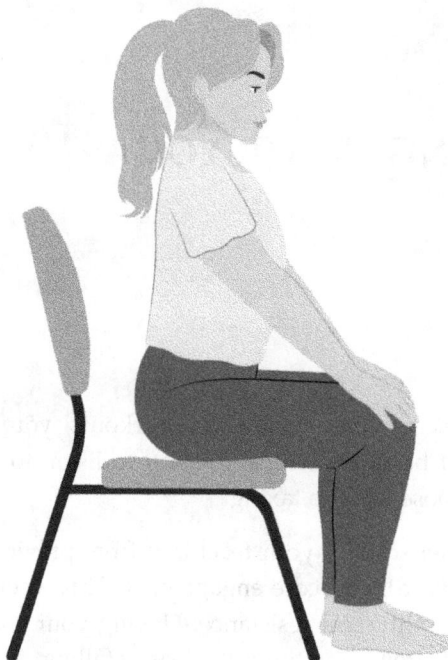

Instructions

- Sit tall in your chair with your feet in front of you, and feet flat on the floor.
- Rest your hands on your knees, palms down, and gaze forward in a neutral position.
- Inhale deeply, and as you exhale, press down into your sitting bones and lengthen your spine.
- As you inhale, engage your core, roll your shoulders back and down, and lift your chest.
- Remain in your mountain pose for 1 minute.

Modifications

- Easier: Use a chair with back support if needed.
- Harder: Close your eyes to increase body awareness.
- Props: Place a folded blanket under your feet if they don't reach the floor.

Tips

- Relax your face and jaw while maintaining the posture.

Seated Revolved Head-to-Knee Pose

This pose stretches the hamstrings, spine, and side body while improving digestion.

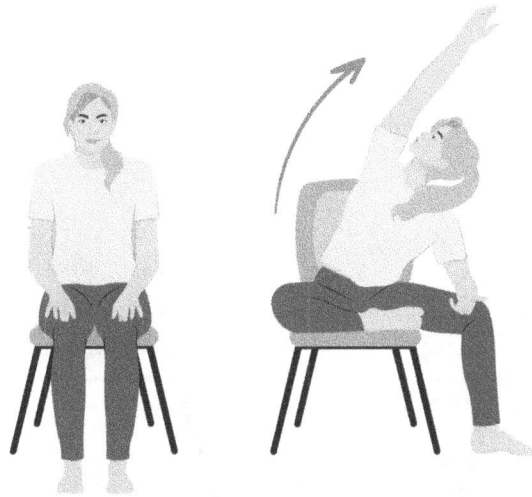

Instructions

- Begin in your neutral mountain pose, feet flat on the floor and your hands on your thighs.
- Inhale and sweep your arms toward the ceiling, palms facing each other.
- Exhale and open your legs to slightly wider than hip-width apart.
- Inhale and lift your left leg, bending at your knee and resting your foot on the seating area with your sole resting on your right thigh.
- Exhale and slowly lower your body to the right, hinging at your hips.
- Drop your right arm to your right thigh for stability and gaze up toward your left hand.
- Hold your pose for 30 seconds.
- Return to center by placing your left leg on the floor and bringing your legs together.
- Place your hands on your thighs to enter your mountain pose.
- Inhale, sweep both arms toward the ceiling, and complete your pose on the other side.

Modifications

- Easier: Keep extended legs bent if hamstrings are tight.
- Harder: Reach for the outer edge of the extended foot with the opposite hand.
- Props: Use a strap around the extended foot if unable to reach it.

Tips

- Keep both sitting bones grounded.
- Twist from your mid-back, not your lower back.
- If you feel knee pain, adjust the bent leg position or come out of the pose.

Seated Extended Hand-to-Big-Toe Pose

This pose stretches the hamstrings, improves balance, and increases flexibility.

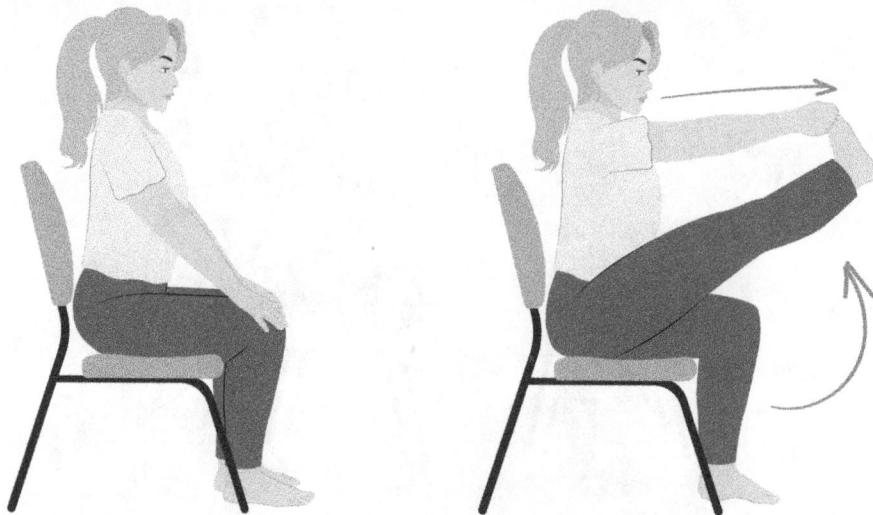

Instructions

- Begin in your neutral mountain pose, feet flat on the floor and your hands on your thighs.
- Inhale deeply and lift your right leg off the floor, straightening your knee.
- Exhale and reach your right hand forward.
- If you can, grab hold of your foot at the toes. Alternatively, use a strap or towel to lengthen your grip.
- Inhale and attempt to sit up tall, straightening your spine.
- Hold your pose for 30 seconds.
- Gradually lower your right foot to the floor and return your hand to your thighs.
- Inhale and lift your left leg off the floor, completing the pose on the other side before returning to your mountain pose.

Modifications

- Easier: Keep the knee slightly bent if the hamstrings are tight.
- Harder: Try to bring the forehead closer to the extended leg.
- Props: Use a yoga strap or towel to reach your feet.

Tips

- Keep your back straight; avoid rounding your spine.
- Engage your quadriceps to help straighten the extended leg.

Chair Side Plank Pose

This pose strengthens the arms, shoulders, and obliques while improving balance.

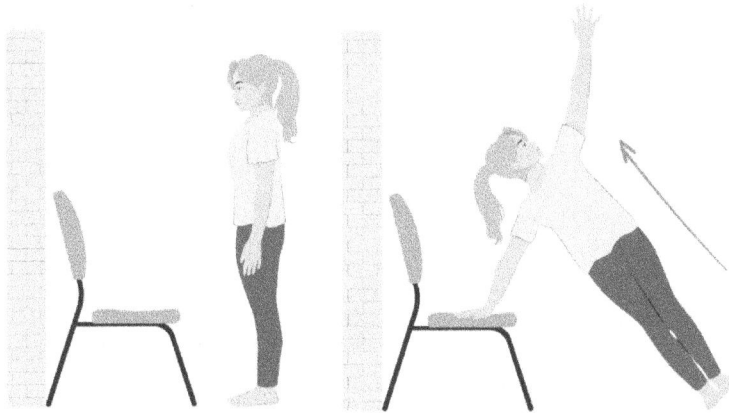

Instructions

- Have the backrest of your chair pushed up against a wall.
- Take a step away from your chair about half an arm's length.
- Inhale, bend your knees slightly, and place both hands on the chair's seating area—ensure your hands are firmly planted and positioned in the middle of your chair.
- Exhale and step back until your legs are straight, your ankles touching, and your spine is straight.
- Inhale and shift your weight onto your right arm. As you do, twist your body, shifting all your weight onto your right arm and leg.
- Ensure your ankles are stacked and that your body is in a straight line.
- Exhale, and as you do, raise your left arm toward the ceiling if you can.
- Hold your pose for 30 seconds.
- To return to your center, place your left foot on the floor, your left hand on the chair, and walk your feet back into a standing position.
- Repeat your pose on the other side.

Modifications

- Easier: Keep the bottom knee on the ground for support.
- Harder: Lift your top leg for an added balance challenge.
- Props: Chair, wall.

Tips

- Keep your supporting arm directly under your shoulder.
- Engage your core to maintain a straight body line.
- If your wrist hurts, make a fist or use yoga blocks on the chair.

Chair Tree Pose

This pose improves balance and focus.

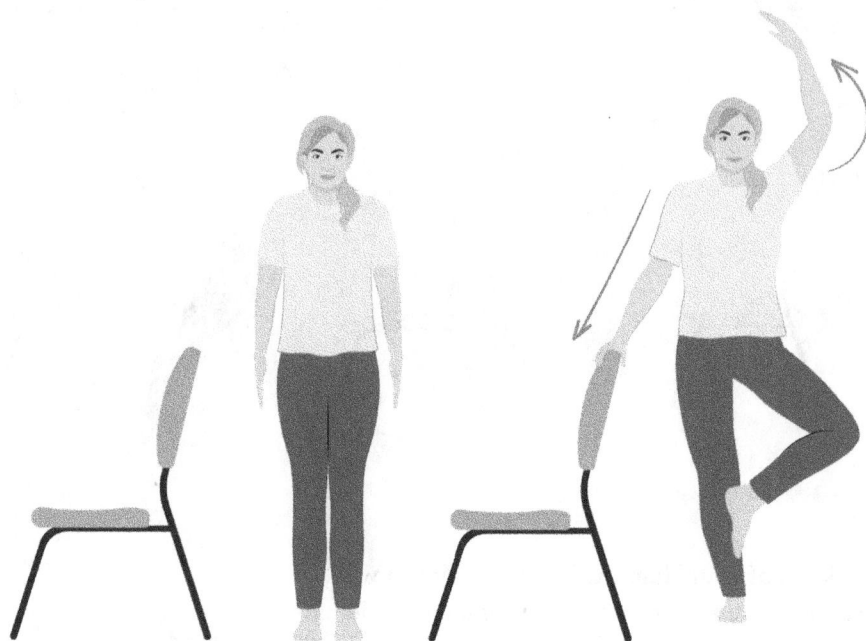

Instructions

- Move your position to the back of your chair and stand with your right side to the backrest.
- Place your right hand on the backrest, inhale, lift your left foot off the floor and engage your core.
- Place the sole of your foot on your calf. Do *not* place your foot on your knee.
- Draw focus to your breath and as you inhale, sweep your left arm up toward the ceiling.
- Keep your elbow slightly bent and your palm facing the ground.
- Gaze forward and hold your pose for 30 seconds.
- Return your left leg to the floor and turn around so your left side faces the backrest.
- Repeat your pose on the other side.

Modifications

- Easier: Keep the raised foot on the ankle instead of the calf.
- Harder: Gaze upward at raised hand.
- Props: Use the chair back for support.

Tips

- Keep your standing leg straight but not locked.
- If you feel unsteady, focus on a fixed point.

Chair Warrior III Pose

This pose strengthens the back and improves balance.

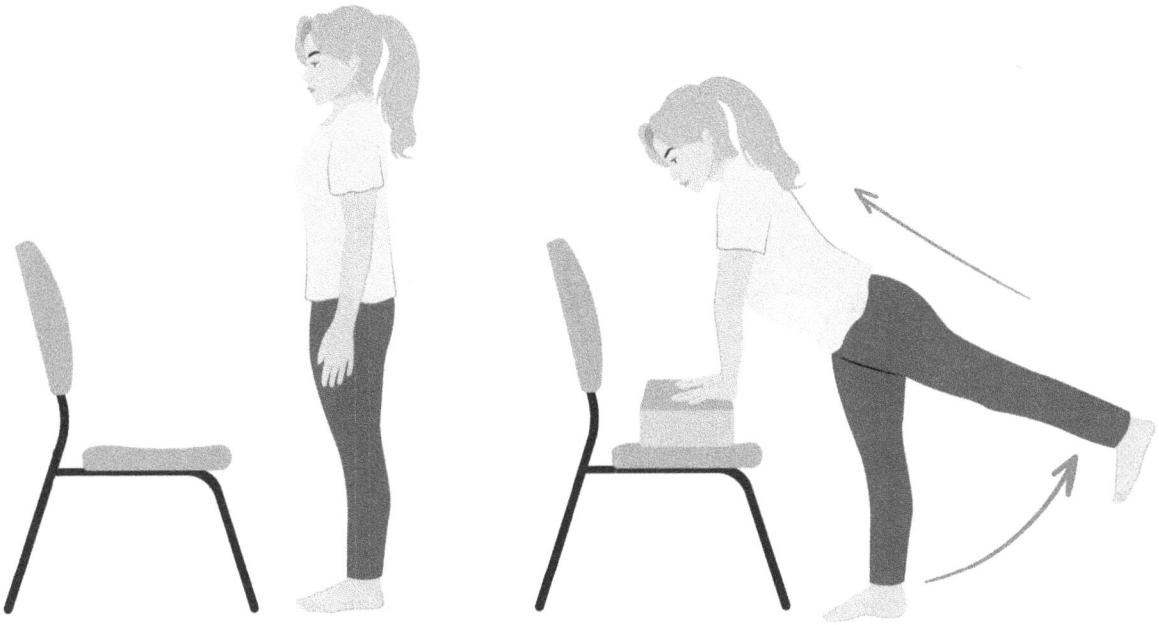

Instructions

- Move to the front of your chair so your body faces the seating area.
- Bring your feet close to the chair and stand tall.
- Inhale, and as you do, lift your right leg off the floor while hinging forward at the hips.
- Drop your hands to the seating area while maintaining a straight line with your spine, and use your right leg for leverage. Gaze down to your hands.
- Hold your pose for 30 seconds.
- Return your right leg to the floor and stand upright.
- Inhale and lift your left leg off the floor to repeat your pose on the other side.

Modifications

- Easier: Keep the standing leg slightly bent.
- Harder: Lift arms parallel to the floor.
- Props: Use blocks on the seat for hand support.

Tips

- Keep hips level throughout the pose.
- Engage core and back muscles.
- Breathe steadily, focusing on balance and alignment.

Chair Crescent Lunge Twist

This pose improves balance, strengthens the legs, and stretches the spine and torso.

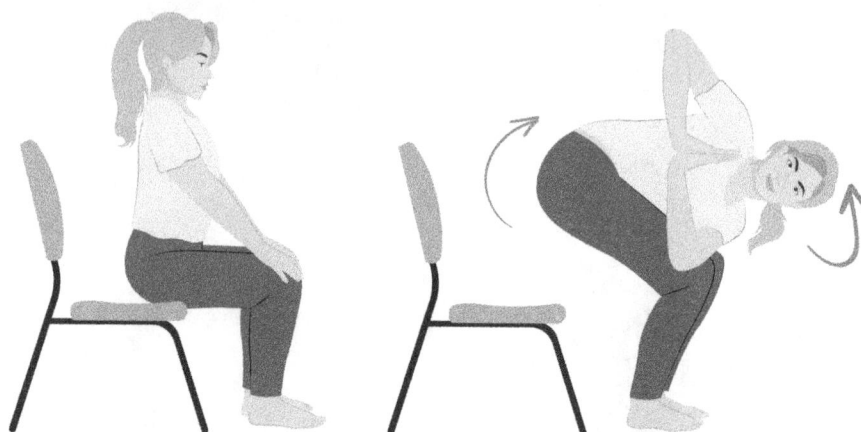

Instructions

- Begin in your neutral mountain pose, feet flat on the floor and your hands resting on your thighs.
- Inhale and sweep your arms above your head, palms facing each other.
- Exhale, and on your next inhale, push through your legs to stand up.
- Bring your ankles together and ensure your feet are facing forward.
- On your next exhale, bend your knees slightly as if you were trying to sit back in your chair—*do not sit.*
- Inhale and bring your hands down to your chest in a prayer position with your elbows bent.
- Exhale and twist your upper body to the right side.
- Hold your pose for 30 seconds.
- Reset your pose by sitting back on your seat and entering the mountain pose.
- Inhale and repeat on the left side before returning to your mountain pose.

Modifications

- Easier: Remain seated while twisting.
- Harder: Lift heels in the standing position.
- Props: Use the chair back for support if needed.

Tips

- Keep feet firmly grounded.
- Engage the core for stability, twisting from your mid-back, not your lower back.
- If you feel any pain, reduce the twist or stop.

Chair Crow Pose

This challenging pose builds arm and core strength while improving balance.

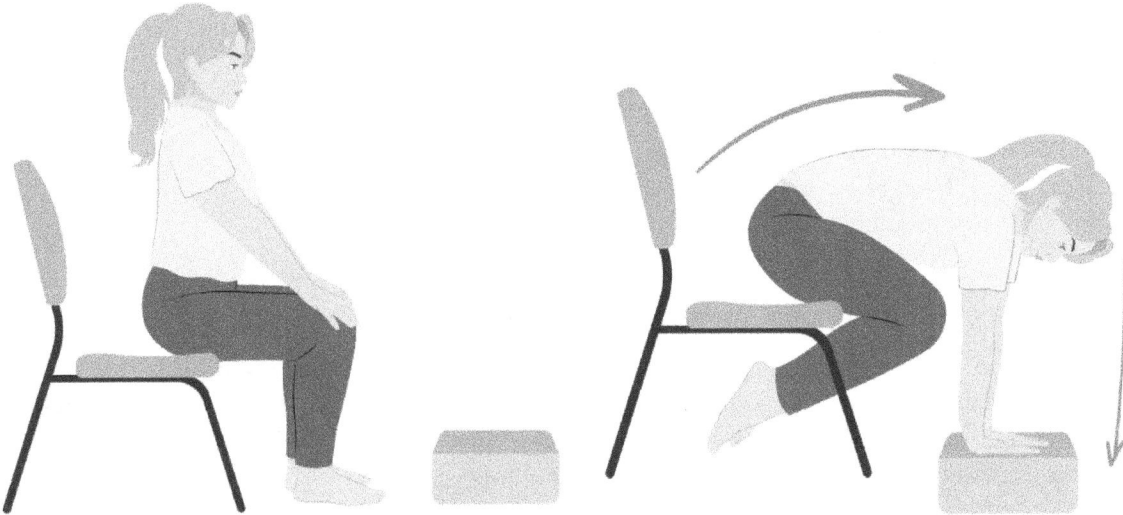

<u>Instructions</u>

- Have the backrest of your chair pushed up against a wall.
- Place a yoga block on the floor in front of your feet's natural position.
- Begin in your neutral mountain pose, feet flat on the floor and your hands on your thighs.
- Focus your breath, and as you inhale, engage your core and lift your feet off the floor.
- Ensure your spine remains straight and that you feel well-balanced.
- Exhale and slowly lower your upper body to the blocks below you.
- Allow your feet to lift and tuck under the seating area of your chair.
- Gaze down toward your hands and keep your spine as straight as possible.
- Hold your pose for 1 minute.

<u>Modifications</u>

- Easier: Keep your toes on the floor for support.
- Harder: Try to hold more of your bodyweight in your arms and off the chair.
- Props: Chair, wall, yoga block.

<u>Tips</u>

- Engage your core throughout the pose for stability.
- Keep your gaze focused on a single point for better balance.
- If you feel unstable, come out of the pose slowly and carefully.

Chair Yoga for Weight Loss: Day 22 to 25

Warm-up: 2 minutes

1. Seated Mountain: 1 minute
2. Chair Revolved Head to Knee: 30 seconds on each side
3. Seated Hand-to-Big-Toe: 30 seconds on each side
4. Chair Side Plank: 30 seconds on each side
5. Chair Tree: 1 minute
6. Chair Warrior III: 30 seconds on each side
7. Chair Crescent Lunge Twist: 30 seconds on each side
8. Chair Crow: 1 minute

The Importance of Nutrition and Hydration

While we've focused primarily on chair yoga's physical and mental aspects, it's important to remember that what you put into your body plays a significant role in your overall wellness and weight loss journey. Proper nutrition and hydration are the foundations upon which we build our health, and they can significantly enhance the benefits of your chair yoga routine.

A balanced diet rich in whole foods provides the energy you need for your chair yoga practice and supports your body's recovery and healing processes. Focus on incorporating a variety of fruits, vegetables, whole grains, lean proteins, and healthy fats into your meals. These foods provide essential vitamins, minerals, and antioxidants that can help reduce inflammation, improve flexibility, and boost overall energy levels.

Pay special attention to foods that support joint health and flexibility, such as:

- Omega-3-rich foods like salmon, walnuts, and flaxseeds
- Colorful fruits and vegetables high in antioxidants
- Protein sources to support muscle repair and growth
- Foods rich in calcium and vitamin D for bone health

There is no one-size-fits-all approach to nutrition. Listen to your body and nourish it with foods that will support lean muscle growth as you become leaner and stronger.

Another important aspect of any wellness journey is proper hydration. Whether we like it or not, water is life, and adequate hydration is crucial for your overall health and yoga practice. Water makes up a significant portion of your body weight and plays a role in nearly every bodily function, including:

- Regulating body temperature
- Transporting nutrients and oxygen to cells
- Cushioning joints
- Removing waste products

When dehydrated, you may experience fatigue, dizziness, and decreased flexibility, which can hinder your chair yoga practice. Aim to drink water consistently throughout the day, not just during your yoga sessions. While individual needs vary, a general guideline is to drink at least 8 glasses (64 ounces) of water per day. You can also get hydration from foods with high water content, such as cucumbers, watermelon, and leafy greens. Herbal teas can be another excellent way to increase fluid intake while providing additional health benefits.

Just as chair yoga encourages mindfulness in movement, try to bring that same awareness to your eating habits. Practice eating slowly, savoring each bite, and paying attention to your body's hunger and fullness cues. This mindful approach to eating can help improve digestion, prevent overeating, and foster a healthier relationship with food.

Day 26-28: Chair Yoga Poses

Five-Pointed Star

This pose strengthens the legs, opens the chest, and improves overall body awareness.

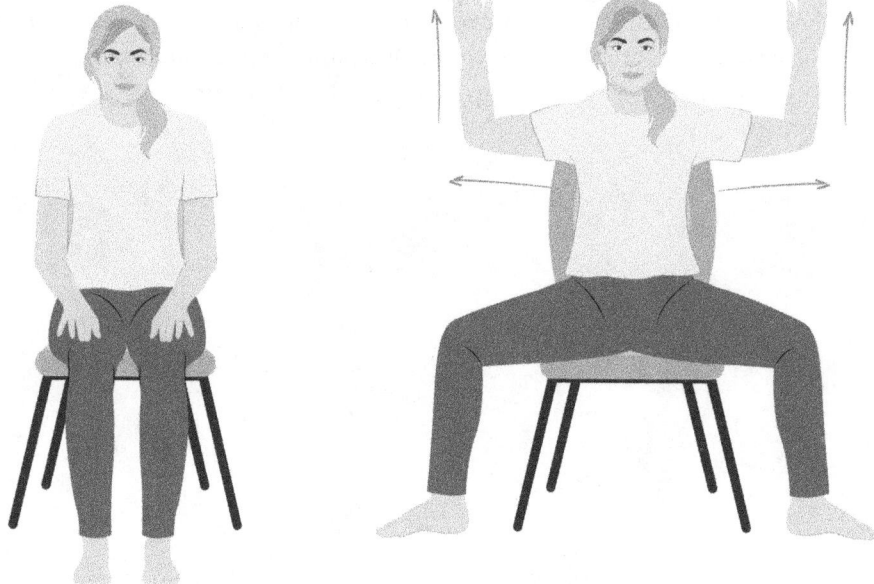

Instructions

- Begin in your neutral mountain pose, feet flat on the floor and your hands on your thighs.
- Inhale and open your legs, widening them to more than hip-width apart.
- Point your toes out at a 45-degree angle and lengthen your spine.
- Exhale and gaze forward.
- Inhale and sweep your arms out to your sides. Keep your elbows straight and your palms facing away from your body.
- Exhale and bend your arms. Spread your fingers wide. Inhale and engage your core.
- Exhale and drop your shoulders back into a relaxed position. Hold your pose for 1 minute.

Modifications

- Easier: Keep arms lower if shoulder mobility is limited.
- Harder: Lift heels off the floor, balancing on toes.
- Props: Use the chair back for support if balance is challenging.

Tips

- Keep your spine straight and chest open throughout the pose.

Wide-Legged Forward Bend

This pose stretches the hamstrings, inner thighs, and lower back.

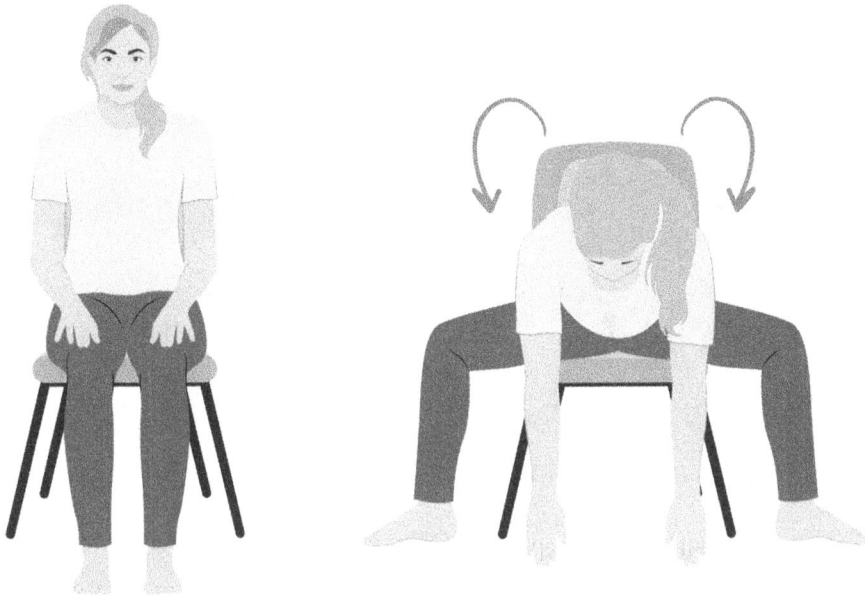

<u>Instructions</u>

- Begin in your neutral mountain pose, feet flat on the floor and your hands on your thighs.
- Inhale and open your legs, widening them to more than hip-width apart.
- Point your toes out at a 45-degree angle and lengthen your spine.
- Exhale and gaze forward.
- Inhale, and as you do, sweep your arms up toward the ceiling. Maintain a forward gaze.
- Exhale and sweep your arms down, hinging at the hips to allow your arms to hang between your legs.
- Inhale and straighten your spine.
- Exhale and press your chest down into the seat of the chair if you can.
- Hold your pose for 1 minute.

<u>Modifications</u>

- Easier: Bend knees slightly if hamstrings are tight.
- Harder: Try to touch the floor with your hands.
- Props: Use yoga blocks to "bring the floor closer."

<u>Tips</u>

- Keep your back straight as you fold forward.
- Engage your quadriceps to protect your hamstrings.

Seated Half Lotus Pose

This pose improves hip flexibility and promotes inner calm.

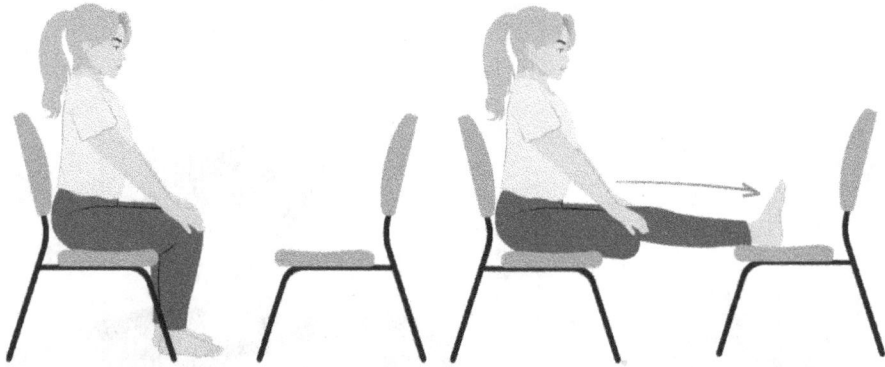

For this pose, you will need an extra chair or sturdy piece of furniture.

<u>Instructions</u>

- Turn your chair so that the seating areas face each other.
- Leave about a chair's width between each chair.
- Begin in neutral mountain pose, feet flat on the floor and hands resting on your thighs.
- Inhale and lift your right leg, bending it at the knee and placing the sole of your foot on your left thigh.
- Exhale and move your hands to your hips, gazing straight ahead.
- Inhale once more and lift your left leg off the floor, straightening it and bringing your heel to rest on the chair in front of you.
- Exhale and lengthen your spine.
- Inhale once more, engage your core and lift your left leg slightly.
- Press your right foot into your left thigh for extra stability, and hold your pose for 30 seconds.
- Release your pose as you exhale, bringing your left and right legs to the floor.
- Place your hands on your thighs to enter into a mountain pose before completing your pose on the other side.

<u>Modifications</u>

- Easier: Keep the bottom foot on the floor if lifting is too challenging.
- Harder: Try to straighten the extended leg more.
- Props: Two chairs or a sturdy piece of furniture.

<u>Tips</u>

- Don't force your foot onto the opposite thigh if it's uncomfortable.
- Keep your spine straight throughout the pose.

Seated Extended Hand-to-Big-Toe Pose

This pose stretches the hamstrings, improves balance, and increases flexibility.

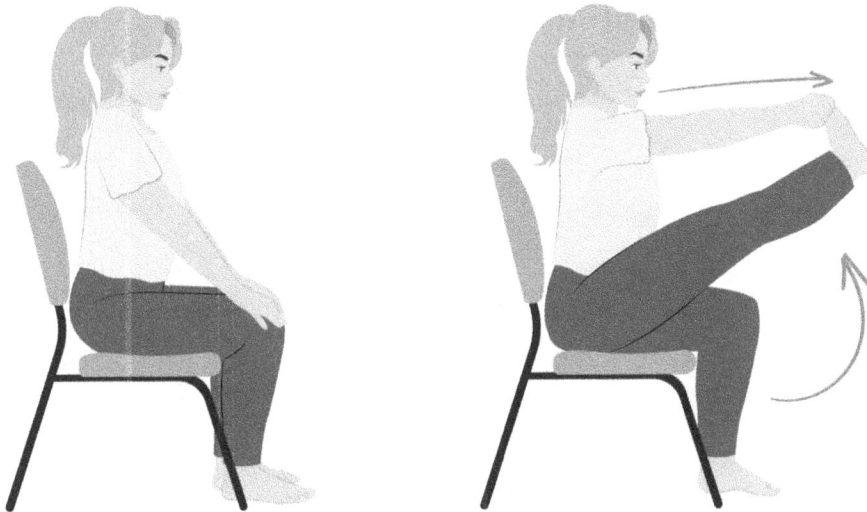

Instructions

- Begin in your neutral mountain pose, feet flat on the floor and your hands resting on your thighs.
- Inhale deeply and lift your right leg off the floor, straightening your knee.
- Exhale and reach your right hand forward.
- If you can, grab hold of your foot at the toes. Alternatively, use a strap or towel to lengthen your grip.
- Inhale and attempt to sit up tall, straightening your spine.
- Hold your pose for 30 seconds.
- Gradually lower your right foot to the floor and return your hand to your thighs.
- Inhale and lift your left leg off the floor, completing the pose on the other side before returning to your mountain pose.

Modifications

- Easier: Keep the knee slightly bent if the hamstrings are tight.
- Harder: Try to bring the forehead closer to the extended leg.
- Props: Use a yoga strap or towel to reach your feet.

Tips

- Keep your back straight; avoid rounding your spine.
- Engage your quadriceps to help straighten the extended leg.

Chair Tree Pose

This pose improves balance and focus.

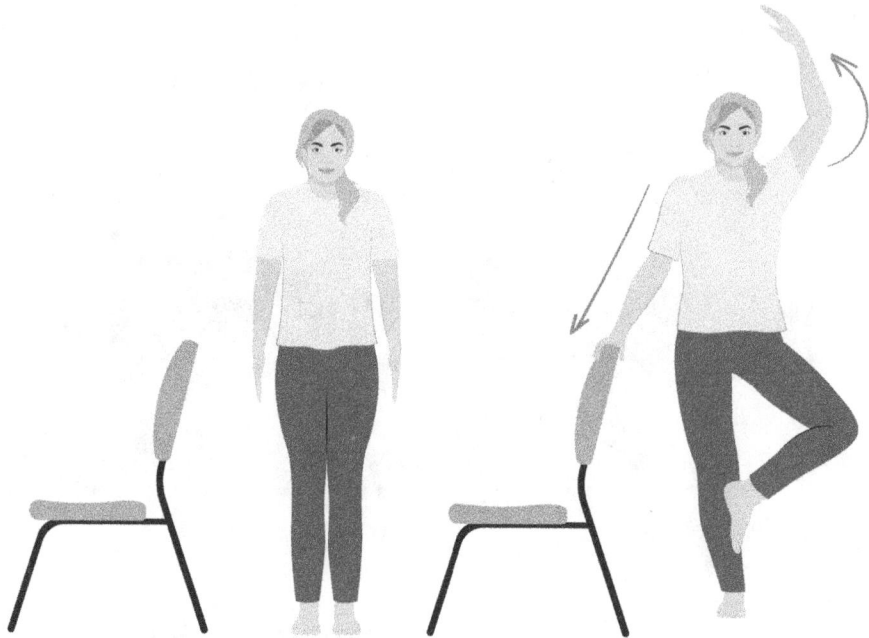

Instructions

- Move your position to the back of your chair and stand with your right side to the backrest.
- Place your right hand on the backrest, inhale, lift your left foot off the floor and engage your core.
- Place the sole of your foot on your calf. Do *not* place your foot on your knee.
- Draw focus to your breath and as you inhale, sweep your left arm up toward the ceiling.
- Keep your elbow slightly bent and your palm facing the ground.
- Gaze forward and hold your pose for 30 seconds.
- Return your left leg to the floor and turn around so your left side faces the backrest.
- Repeat your pose on the other side.

Modifications

- Easier: Keep the raised foot on the ankle instead of the calf.
- Harder: Gaze upward at raised hand.
- Props: Use the chair back for support.

Tips

- Keep your standing leg straight but not locked.
- If you feel unsteady, focus on a fixed point.

Chair Bound Revolved Half Moon Pose

This advanced pose improves balance, strengthens the legs and core, and increases hip and spine flexibility.

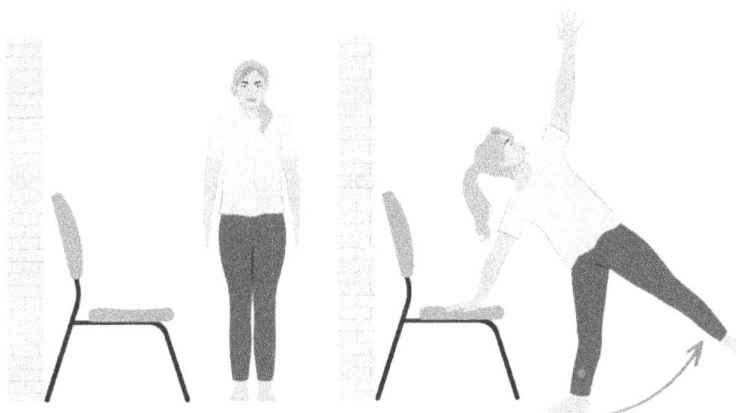

Instructions

- Have the backrest of your chair pushed up against a wall.
- Stand with your right hip facing the seating area of the chair.
- Take a step away from your chair about half an arm's length.
- Inhale, and as you do, drop your right hand to the seating area.
- Gradually lift your left leg off the floor, aiming to hold it at a 45-degree angle (no higher or lower).
- Exhale and adjust your right foot so your toes point toward the chair slightly.
- Inhale and sweep your left hand toward the ceiling, aiming to form a straight line with your right arm.
- Gaze over your left shoulder and hold your pose for 30 seconds.
- Place your left foot flat on the floor and hinge your hips to stand upright.
- Repeat on the other side.

Modifications

- Easier: Keep the raised leg's foot on the floor for balance.
- Harder: Try to raise the leg higher, closer to parallel with the floor.
- Props: Chair, wall for support.

Tips

- Keep the standing leg slightly bent to protect the knee.
- Engage your core for stability and balance.
- If balance is challenging, focus your gaze on a fixed point.

Chair Side Plank Pose

This pose strengthens the arms, shoulders, and obliques while improving balance.

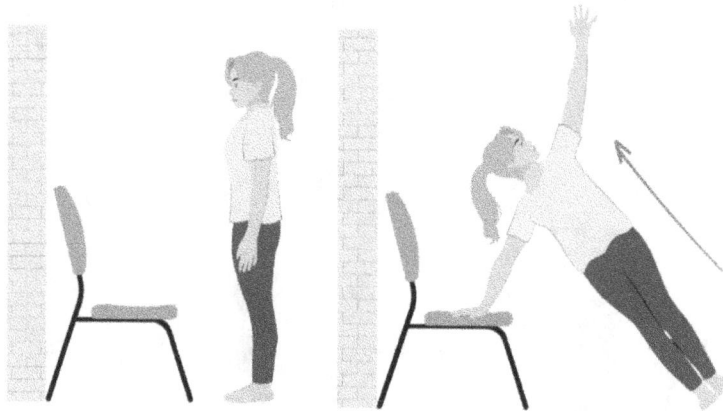

Instructions

- Have the backrest of your chair pushed up against a wall.
- Stand facing your chair's seating area.
- Take a step away from your chair about half an arm's length.
- Inhale, bend your knees slightly, and place both hands on the chair's seating area—ensure your hands are firmly planted and positioned in the middle of your chair.
- Exhale and step back until your legs are straight, your ankles touching, and your spine is straight.
- Inhale and shift your weight onto your right arm. As you do, twist your body, shifting all your weight onto your right arm and leg.
- Ensure your ankles are stacked and that your body is in a straight line.
- Exhale, and as you do, raise your left arm toward the ceiling if you can.
- Hold your pose for 30 seconds.
- To return to your center, place your left foot on the floor, your left hand on the chair, and walk your feet back into a standing position.
- Repeat your pose on the other side.

Modifications

- Easier: Keep the bottom knee on the ground for support.
- Harder: Lift your top leg for an added balance challenge.
- Props: Chair, wall.

Tips

- Keep your supporting arm directly under your shoulder.
- Engage your core to maintain a straight body line.

Chair Crow Pose

This challenging pose builds arm and core strength while improving balance.

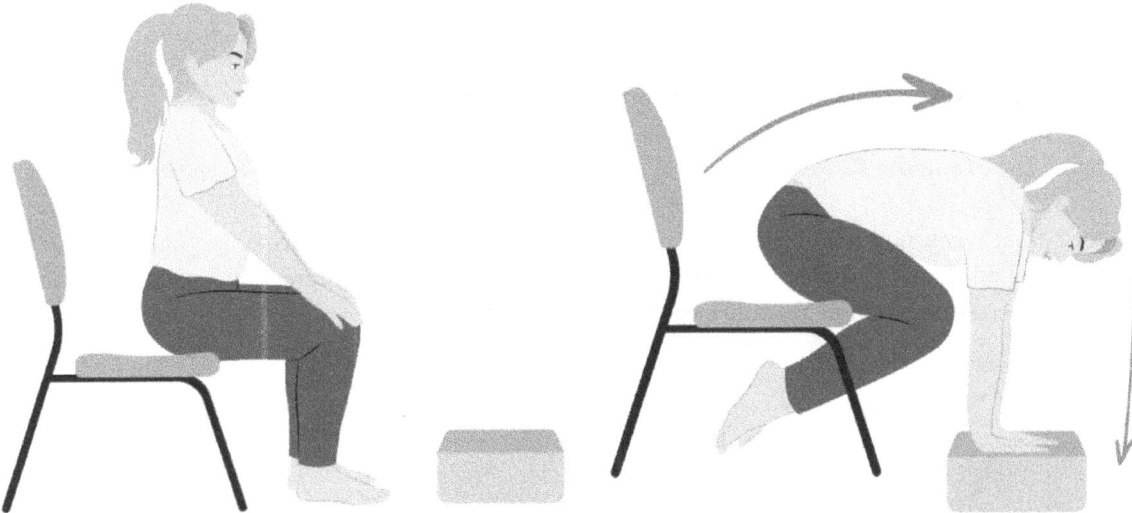

Instructions

- Have the backrest of your chair pushed up against a wall.
- Place a yoga block on the floor in front of your feet's natural position.
- Begin in your neutral mountain pose, feet flat on the floor and your hands on your thighs.
- Focus your breath, and as you inhale, engage your core and lift your feet off the floor.
- Ensure your spine remains straight and that you feel well-balanced.
- Exhale and slowly lower your upper body to the blocks below you.
- Allow your feet to lift and tuck under the seating area of your chair.
- Gaze down toward your hands and keep your spine as straight as possible.
- Hold your pose for 1 minute.
- To come out of your pose, place your feet on the floor, hinge at the hips, and sit upright.

Modifications

- Easier: Keep your toes on the floor for support.
- Harder: Try to hold more of your bodyweight in your arms and off the chair.
- Props: Chair, wall, yoga block.

Tips

- Engage your core throughout the pose for stability.
- Keep your gaze focused on a single point for better balance.

Chair Yoga for Weight Loss: Day 26 to 28

1. Seated Five-Pointed Star: 1 minute
2. Seated Wide-Legged Forward Bend: 1 minute
3. Seated Half Lotus: 1 minute
4. Seated Revolved Hand-to-Big-Toe: 30 seconds on each side
5. Chair Tree: 1 minute
6. Chair Bound Revolved Half Moon: 30 seconds on each side
7. Chair Side Plank: 30 seconds on each side
8. Chair Crow: 1 minute

With your final week now complete, we must explore your chair yoga journey beyond these 28 days. Before moving on to this next chapter, take a moment to celebrate your progress and your commitment to creating a leaner, stronger, more flexible body, one yoga pose at a time.

CHAPTER 8

BEYOND THE 28 DAYS—INTEGRATING CHAIR YOGA INTO YOUR LIFESTYLE

*T*he end of your 28-day challenge is by no means the end of your chair yoga journey, nor should it be the end of your pursuit of health and well-being. Your body has become stronger and more flexible and may be ready for more challenging workouts. If you're not quite ready, that's perfectly fine as well.

While 28 days does not sound like a significant period of time, your perseverance has benefited your body, even if the scale has not moved. Now is the time to anchor down, commit to your health, and build a strong, capable body.

Integrating chair yoga into your daily life has shown you the power of consistency and how capable your body is. Moving forward from your structured chair yoga workout, you must create a solid foundation for further development and growth. Here's how.

- **Set realistic goals and expectations for yourself**. Remember, your workouts are practice and do not demand perfection. Some days, you may have extra time on your hands to do another workout or a longer warmup; others, you will only have 10 minutes to spare; and some days, you may not have time. What is important is to show up for yourself with kindness and compassion.
- **Create a dedicated space for your practice so that you can focus on your workouts**. This could be a corner of your bedroom or a spot in your office—whatever works. Having a physical space allows you to disengage from all of the other activities you need to get done so that you can focus on yourself for 10 minutes.
- **Experiment with different styles of yoga and, specifically, chair yoga**. Just like no two bodies are exactly alike, no two chair yoga practices will be either. Don't be afraid to try different poses, sequences, and even teachers to find what resonates with you and your unique needs and goals.
- **Find a community**. I can't emphasize enough how important it is to integrate into a community that loves and supports each other to keep going. You don't have to physically go somewhere to meet like-minded people anymore (although you absolutely can if that is what you want). Check out online chair yoga and social media groups dedicated to at-home chair yoga practitioners.

- **Keep the bigger picture in mind**. Chair yoga is about so much more than just the physical poses. It's about cultivating a deeper sense of awareness, compassion, and resilience—both on and off the chair. So, as you continue to integrate this practice into your life, remember to approach it with curiosity, openness, and gratitude for all the ways it's already supporting and transforming you.
- **Explore complementary practices like meditation, breathwork, and self-care to round out your holistic wellness routine**. These practices help to regulate your nervous system further, lowering cortisol and improving your body's natural fat-burning capabilities.
- **Listen to your body**. Create your own practice and flow of movements beyond these routines.

Chair Yoga Prop Guide

While technology can be useful in tracking your progress, you shouldn't overlook the power of simple tools to enhance your chair yoga practice.

Yoga straps, blocks, pillows, and even a simple notebook and pen may be tremendously helpful in both your practice and your broader quest for well-being. While we have already discussed some props you can use and alternatives to them, it's important to understand how effective these can be in deepening your practice.

When Do You Need Props?

Consider investing in props when:

- You're just starting out and need extra support.
- You have limited flexibility or mobility.
- You want to deepen your practice and explore more challenging variations of poses.
- You're recovering from an injury and need to modify your practice.

What to Look for When Buying Props

1. Yoga Blocks

- Material: Foam blocks are lightweight and affordable, while cork or wood blocks are more durable and stable.
- Size: Standard blocks are 9" x 6" x 4", but smaller sizes are available if you have smaller hands.

2. Yoga Straps

- Length: 6-foot straps are versatile for most uses, but longer straps (8-10 feet) offer more options.
- Material: Look for durable cotton or nylon straps with a secure buckle.

3. Bolsters

- Firmness: Choose a bolster that's firm enough to provide support but soft enough for comfort.
- Shape: Cylindrical bolsters are versatile, while rectangular ones are great for restorative poses.

4. Blankets

- Material: Mexican yoga blankets are traditional, but any firm, non-slip blanket will do.
- Thickness: Thicker blankets provide more support and cushioning.

Where to Buy Props

- Local yoga studios often sell high-quality props and can offer personalized advice.
- Sporting goods stores typically have a yoga section with a variety of props.
- Online retailers offer a wide selection, often at competitive prices. Just be sure to read reviews before purchasing.

Ultimately, your journey beyond 28 days is what you want to make of it. Whether that means building your own community, integrating complimentary practices, or venturing off the chair to try new modalities is up to you.

There is no right or wrong way to continue your weight loss journey—it simply requires consistency and your ability to remain open, curious, and compassionate.

A Gift for You

To support you in your chair yoga for weight loss journey, we have put together a *Chair Yoga 3 in 1 Journal*. This invaluable tool allows you to keep track of your progress, gain access to daily insights, and take advantage of planning your meals ahead of time for the entire 28 days of your program.

Simply scan the QR code below or click the url link to access to your *Chair Yoga Journal*.

https://drive.google.com/file/d/11XMb_BkQG1F5WXVH5G8X0kPZs1C6OHBK/view?usp=drive_link

CHAPTER 9
BONUS POSES

These bonus poses include alternative poses, some considered advanced and will test your balance and strength. It is *not* recommended that you attempt these poses until you understand the poses well in weeks 1 through 4.

Seated Ankle Circles

This pose mobilizes the ankles and feet, reducing stiffness and improving circulation.

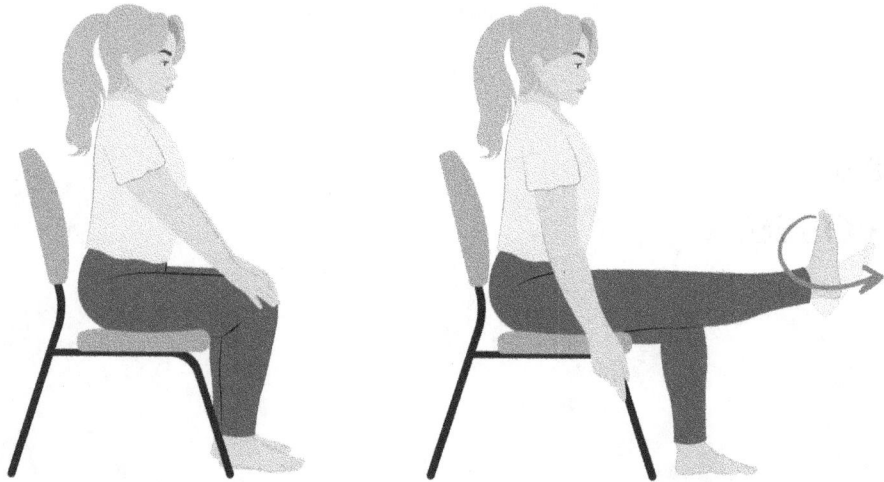

Instructions

- From your mountain pose, bring both hands to your right thigh.
- Inhale, and as you do, lift your left foot off the floor.
- Exhale and circle your left ankle in clockwise movements for 15 seconds.
- Draw focus to your breath. On your next exhale, rotate your ankle counterclockwise for 15 seconds.
- Place your foot back on the ground and place both hands on your left thigh.
- Lift your right foot off the ground and repeat the exercises in both a clockwise and counterclockwise direction.
- Return to your mountain pose.

Modifications

- Easier: Keep your foot closer to the ground if extending your leg is challenging.
- Harder: Point and flex your foot as you circle to engage more muscles.
- Props: None required.

Tips

- Keep your leg as still as possible, isolating the movement to your ankle.
- Make the circles as large as comfortably possible.
- If you experience pain or clicking in your ankle, reduce the range of motion or stop.

Chair Pigeon Pose

This deeper version of the figure four pose pose stretches the hips, glutes, and lower back, helping to relieve tension and improve flexibility.

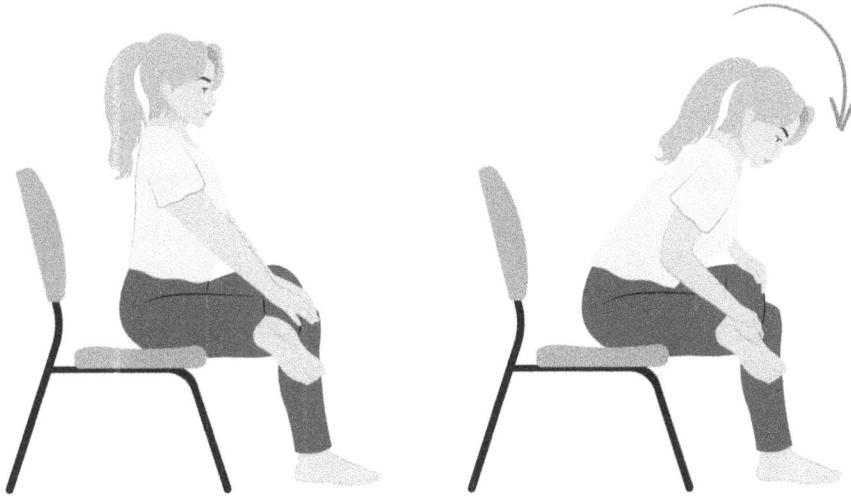

Instructions

- Begin in your neutral mountain pose, feet flat on the floor and your hands on your thighs.
- As you inhale, lift your right leg, bend your knee, and place your right ankle on your left thigh.
- Place one hand on your right knee and one on your right ankle for stability.
- Keep your spine long and straight and your gaze forward.
- On your next exhale, hinge forward at the hips, lowering your torso towards your thighs.
- Pull on your leg for a deeper stretch.
- Hold the pose for 30 seconds.
- Return to your center by returning your right foot to the floor.
- On your next inhale, lift your left leg, bend at the knee, and repeat your pose.
- Return to your mountain pose.

Modifications

- Easier: Keep your torso upright if folding forward is too intense.
- Harder: Reach for your left foot with both hands in the forward fold.
- Props: Place a cushion under your raised foot for support if needed.

Tips

- Keep your spine straight, even as you fold forward.
- Don't force your knee down; let it open naturally.
- If you feel any pain in your knee or hip, reduce the stretch or stop.

Standing Forward Lunge

This pose strengthens the legs, improves balance, and stretches the hip flexors.

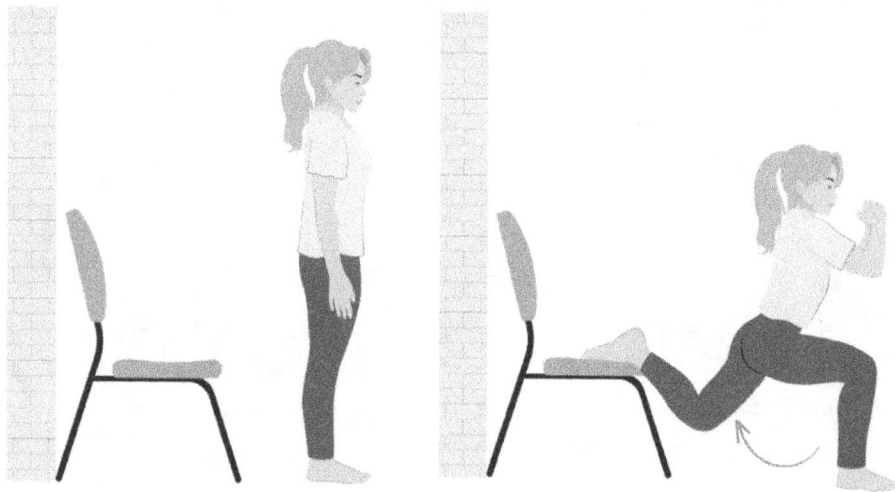

Instructions

- Have the back of the chair against a wall, and turn around so that your back is to the chair.
- Inhale and lift your right foot, bending the knee and placing your foot on the chair's seat.
- Exhale and bring your hands to your chest in a prayer position.
- Inhale and take a step forward with your left leg, using your right foot for balance.
- Exhale and bend your right knee, entering into a lunge position.
- Inhale and straighten your spine, ensuring a straight line runs from the crown of your head down to your right knee.
- Hold your pose for 30 seconds.
- To release your pose, straighten your left leg, place your right foot back on the floor, and step back to your starting position.
- Now, inhale and lift your left foot, bending at the knee and placing your foot on the seat.
- Repeat your pose on the other side.
- Place your left foot back on the floor and return to a neutral standing position with your back facing your chair.

Modifications

- Easier: Keep your back knee on the chair seat.
- Harder: Raise arms overhead in the lunge.
- Props: Chair and wall for balance if needed.

Tips

- Keep the front knee aligned over the ankle.

Seated Tricep Dip

This pose strengthens the triceps, shoulders, and chest.

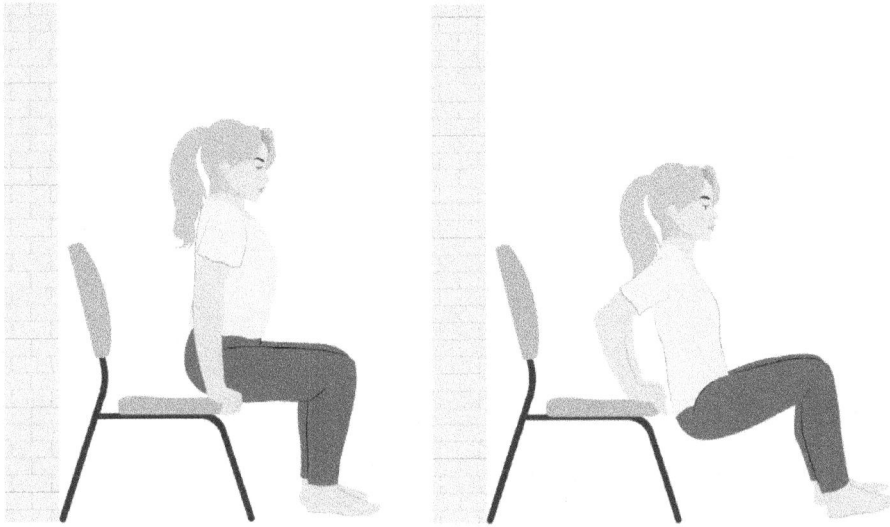

Instructions

- Have the backrest of your chair pushed up against a wall.
- From your standing position, sit on the very edge of your chair.
- Place your hands on the front of your seating area facing forward.
- Bend your knees, lengthen your spine, and gaze forward.
- Inhale, and as you do, lift your behind off the chair.
- Ground yourself using your feet and ensure your arms support your body weight.
- Exhale and lower your upper body off the chair. Bend at your elbows and lift your toes off the floor so that your hands and heels support your weight.
- Hold your pose for 1 minute.
- To return to neutral position, push through your arms, straighten your legs, and sit back.

Modifications

- Easier: Keep your feet flat on the floor throughout.
- Harder: Extend legs straight out in front.
- Props: Chair, wall.

Tips

- Keep shoulders down, away from ears.
- Engage the core throughout the pose.
- If you feel any shoulder pain, come out of the pose.

Raised Glute Bridge

This pose strengthens the glutes, hamstrings, and lower back.

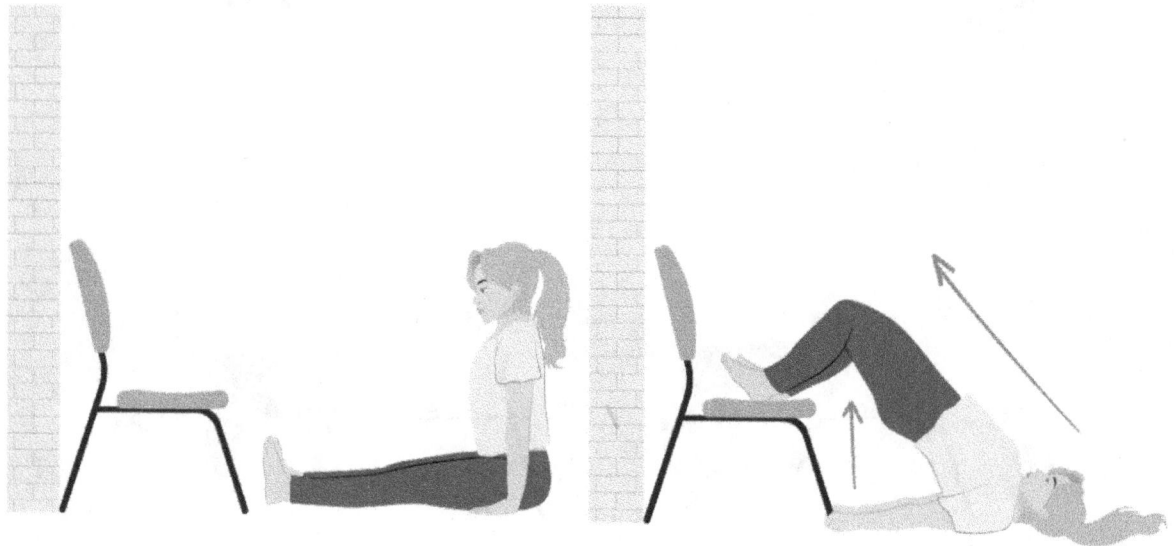

Instructions

- Have the backrest of your chair pushed up against a wall.
- From your seated position on the floor, place your hands at your sides and lengthen your spine.
- Inhale, engage your core and lie back so your back is flat on the floor.
- Exhale and place both feet on the seating area of your chair.
- Bend your knees and reposition your upper body so that your hands can grab hold of the front legs of your chair.
- Inhale deeply, and as you do, push through your feet to lift your lower body off the floor.
- Straighten your spine so that your thighs and spine form a straight line.
- Hold your pose for 1 minute.

Modifications

- Easier: Keep hips lower if full extension is challenging.
- Harder: Lift one foot off the chair seat for a single-leg bridge.
- Props: Chair, wall.

Tips

- Keep shoulders pressed into the floor.
- Engage the core throughout the pose.
- If you feel any strain in the lower back, lower your hips slightly.

Chair Revolved Hand-to-Big-Toe Pose

This pose improves flexibility in the hamstrings and hips while challenging balance.

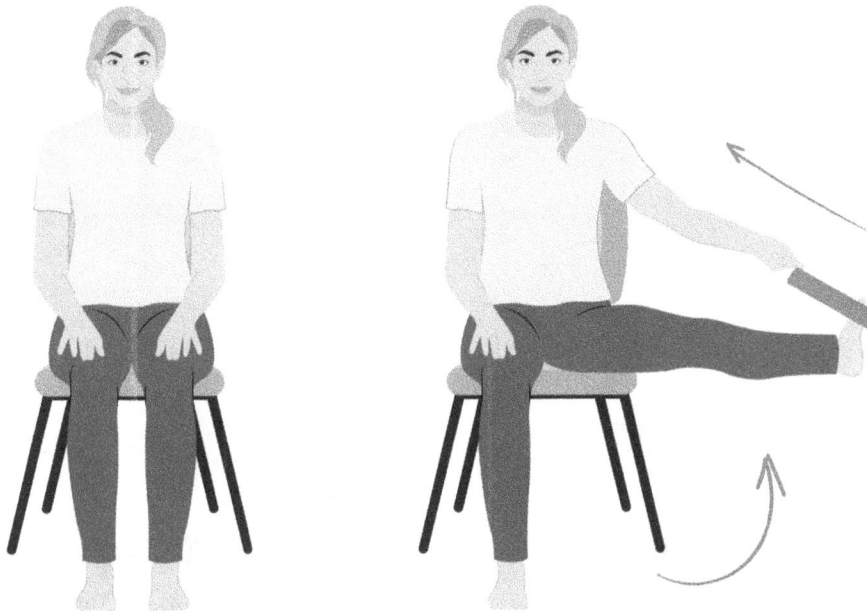

Instructions

- Begin in your neutral mountain pose, feet flat on the floor and your hands on your thighs.
- Inhale, and as you do, straighten your right leg and lift it straight out in front of you.
- Exhale and lean forward to grab hold of your foot.
- Inhale once more, and using your hand, guide your right leg out to your right side.
- Exhale, and as you do, try to sit your upper body up straight.
- Hold your pose for 30 seconds.
- To release your pose, lower your right leg to the floor and enter the mountain pose.
- Inhale deeply, straighten your left leg, lifting it off the floor to repeat your pose on the other side.

Modifications

- Easier: Use a strap around the foot if you can't reach it.
- Harder: Try to bring the leg closer to the torso.
- Props: Yoga strap if needed.

Tips

- Keep your sit bones grounded on the chair.
- If your hamstrings are tight, keep a slight bend in the extended leg.
- Focus on lengthening the spine as you hold the pose.

Seated Forward Bend with Twist

This pose combines a forward bend with a twist, stretching the back, hamstrings, and sides of the body.

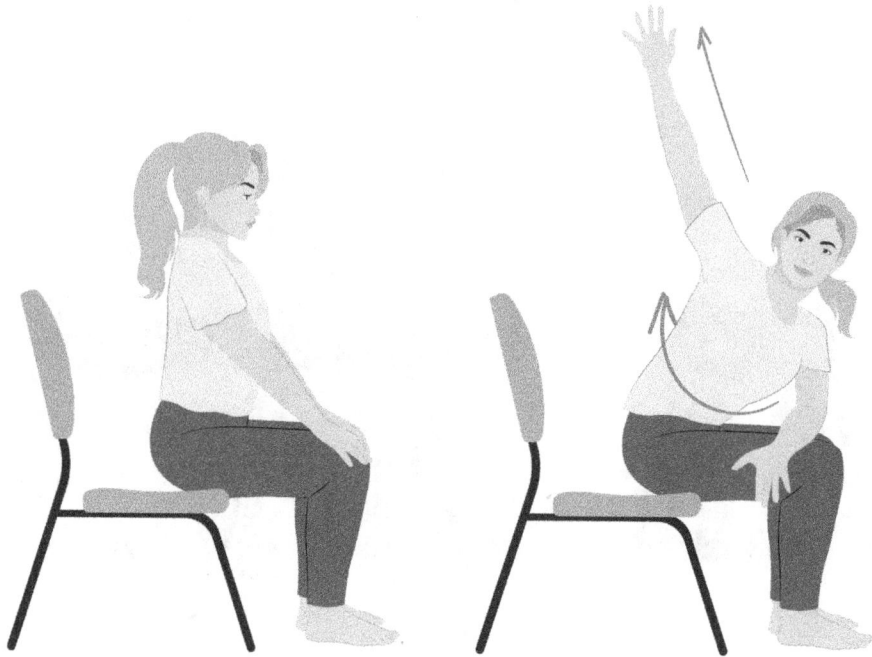

Instructions

- Begin in your neutral mountain pose, feet flat on the floor and your hands on your thighs.
- Inhale deeply, and as you do, sweep your hands straight up above your head.
- Keep your arms straight and your palms facing each other.
- Exhale and drop your right shoulder, twisting your upper body to the left.
- Bend your right elbow and rest your forearm on your thighs, gaze over your left shoulder.
- Inhale once more and lower your chest to your thighs.
- Hold your pose for 30 seconds.
- Return to your center by dropping your left arm and sitting upright in your mountain pose.
- Exhale, drop your left shoulder, and repeat your pose on the other side.

Modifications

- Easier: Twist less deeply if flexibility is limited.
- Harder: Try to bring the chest closer to the thighs in the forward bend.
- Props: Use a strap around your feet if your hands don't reach in a forward bend.

Tips

- Twist from your mid-back, not your lower back.

Standing Half-Plank

This pose strengthens the arms, shoulders, and core while improving overall body alignment.

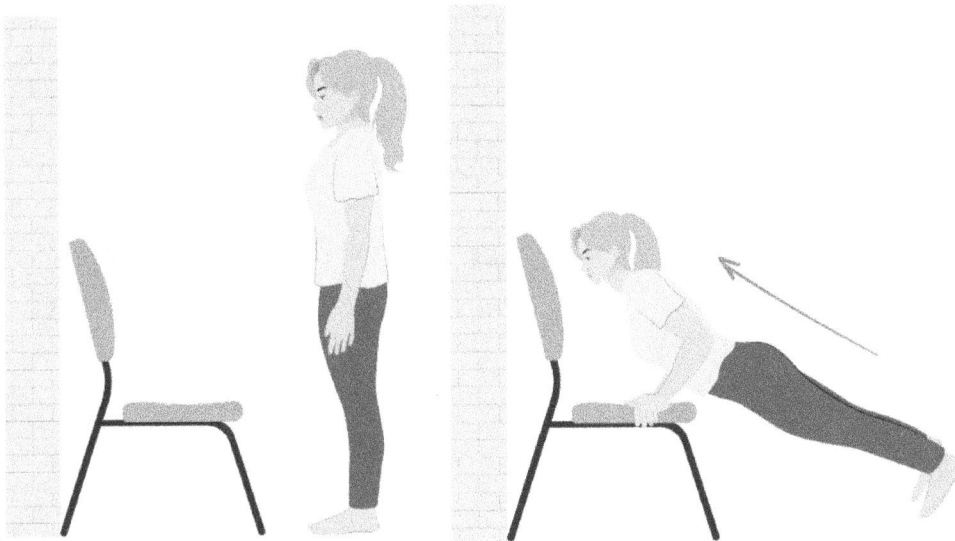

Instructions

- Have the backrest of your chair pushed up against a wall.
- Stand tall, facing your chair.
- Inhale deeply and sweep your arms up toward the ceiling.
- Exhale and bring your hands down, placing them on either side of your seating area.
- Bend your elbows and gaze forward over the seating area.
- Inhale and take a big step back with your dominant foot first and then your non-dominant foot.
- Straighten your legs, push through your toes, and engage your abdominal muscles to maintain a straight line from your head to your toes.
- Keep your elbows bent and your gaze forward.
- Hold your pose for 1 minute.

Modifications

- Easier: Keep your knees on the floor for less intensity.
- Harder: Straighten arms for full plank position.
- Props: Chair, wall.

Tips

- Keep the body in a straight line from head to heels.
- Engage the core throughout the pose.

Chair Wheel Pose

This pose opens the chest, strengthens the back, and improves spinal flexibility.

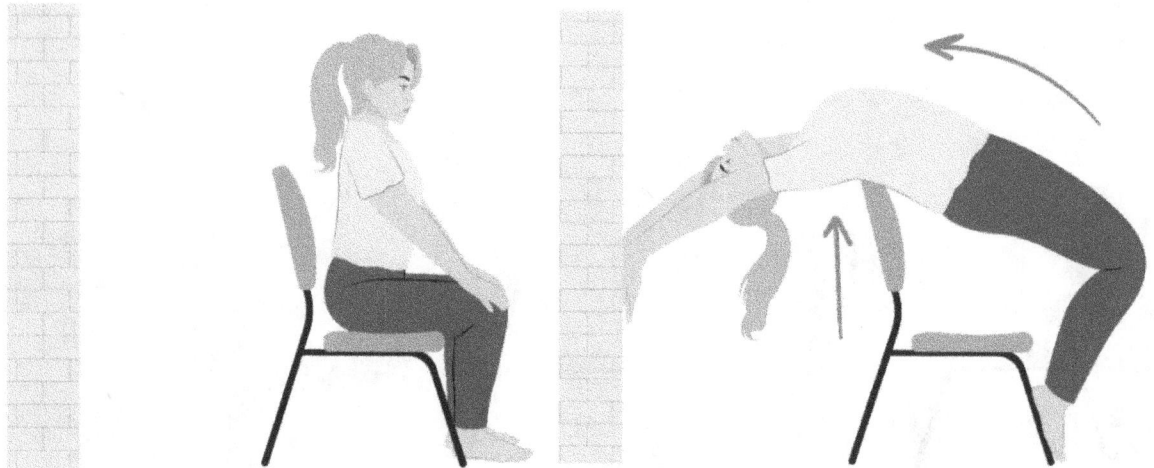

Instructions

- Have the backrest of your chair about 4 inches from the wall.
- Sit on the very edge of your chair, placing your hands on your thighs and your feet against the front legs of your chair.
- Inhale, and sweep your arms back over your head.
- Allow your body to lift off your chair by pushing up through your legs.
- If you can, place your hands on the wall and arch your upper back over the backrest of the chair to deepen your "wheel" position.
- Hold your pose for 30 seconds.
- To release, straighten your back, place your behind on the seating area, and sit upright.

Modifications

- Easier: Keep hips on the chair; just arch the upper back.
- Harder: Try to lift hips higher, creating deeper backbends.
- Props: Chair, wall.

Tips

- Warm up back thoroughly before this pose.
- Keep your neck in line with your spine; don't drop your head back.
- If you feel any pinching in the lower back, come out of the pose.

Seated Child's Pose

This restorative pose helps release tension in the back, shoulders, and neck.

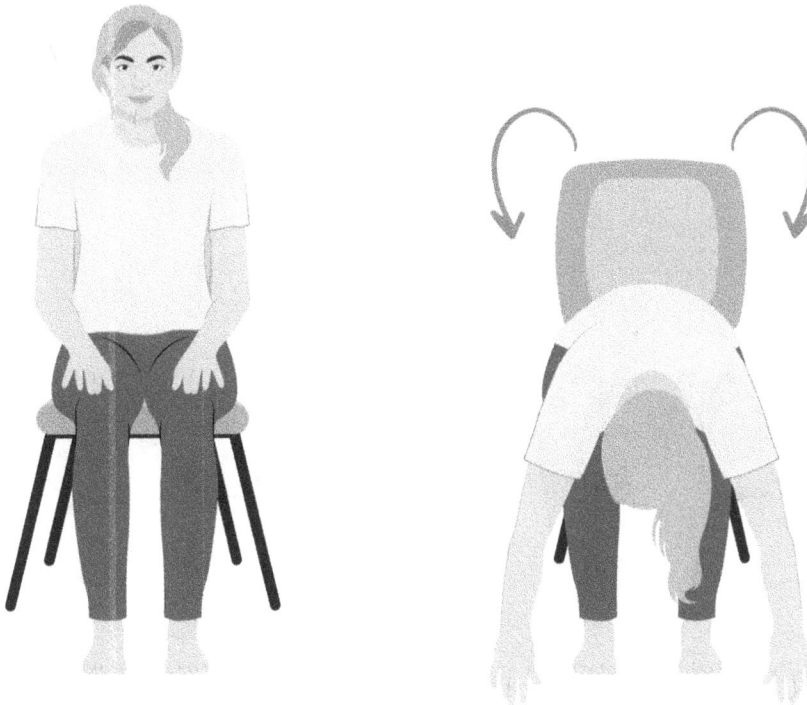

<u>Instructions</u>

- Begin in your neutral mountain pose, feet flat on the floor and your hands on your thighs.
- Widen your legs so they are on either side of the chair.
- Inhale deeply, and as you do, sweep your hands straight up above your head.
- Keep your arms straight and your palms facing each other.
- Exhale and fold forward at your hips, allowing your arms to hang in front of you.
- Allow your head to hang comfortably and freely.

<u>Modifications</u>

- Easier: Place a cushion on your lap to rest your forehead.
- Harder: Reach arms further forward on the ground.
- Props: Cushion or folded blanket for support.

<u>Tips</u>

- Let gravity do the work—don't force the forward bend.
- Relax your neck and shoulders completely.

Seated Relaxation Pose

This pose helps release tension in the lower back and promotes relaxation.

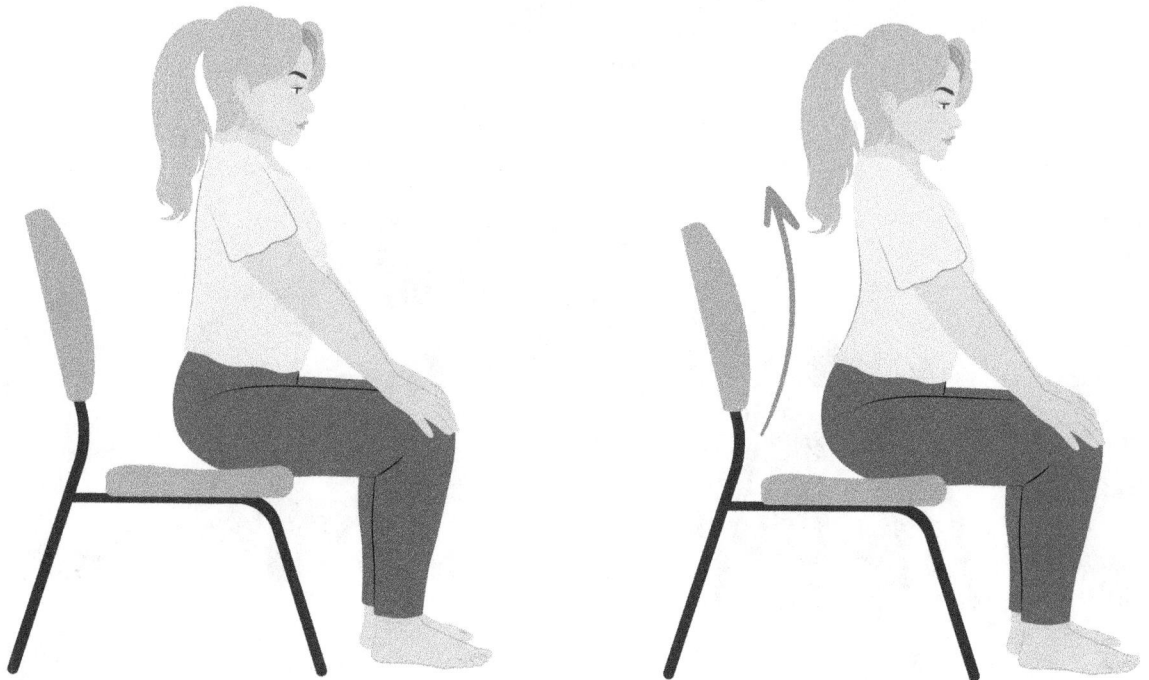

Instructions

- Begin in your neutral mountain pose, feet flat on the floor and your hands on your thighs.
- Inhale deeply, and as you do, arch your mid-back, pushing your shoulders and pelvis back and forming an arch with your lower back.
- Exhale and drop your hands to the bottom of your knees.
- Inhale and fix your gaze forward.
- Hold your pose for as long as you like.

Modifications

- Easier: Use the chair back for support if needed.
- Harder: Try to increase the arch in your lower back.
- Props: None required.

Tips

- Don't force the arch; go only as far as is comfortable.
- Keep your feet flat on the floor for grounding.

CONCLUSION

As we conclude your transformative chair yoga weight loss journey, take a moment to reflect on how far you've come. From those initial gentle seated twists to more challenging flows, you've developed and grown far beyond poses in a chair. This weight loss journey has been about discovering your own route to wellness, building resilience, adapting to life's challenges, and unlocking your boundless potential for growth and change. With every workout, you've demonstrated that positive transformation is possible and achievable when you commit to yourself.

Chair yoga has revealed itself as more than just an exercise routine—it's a lifestyle that nurtures presence, compassion, and self-connection in every moment. This practice taught you to honor your body as a sacred vessel deserving of love and care. You've uncovered that genuine strength and flexibility stem not from physical prowess but from consistently prioritizing yourself and your health with courage, humor, and an open heart. Perhaps most importantly, chair yoga has reaffirmed your inherent worth and capacity for joy, regardless of life's circumstances.

Let's revisit why chair yoga is such a powerful tool for improving your health and supporting weight loss. It's a low-impact method to boost your heart rate and increase movement, helping burn calories and rev up your metabolism over time. Plus, it's far more enjoyable than trudging on a treadmill! Chair yoga builds strength and tones muscles, especially in often-neglected areas like your core, arms, and legs. You've likely noticed improved flexibility and range of motion, reducing pain, stiffness, and injury risk both on and off the chair.

As a fantastic stress-buster, chair yoga is crucial for overall health and weight management. Instead of reaching for comfort food when stressed, it offers a healthier coping mechanism. By increasing body awareness and mindfulness, chair yoga helps you tune into your body's cues, leading to more intuitive choices about food and self-care. The chair yoga community provides invaluable support and connection, essential for sustained motivation on your wellness journey. And remember, it's accessible and adaptable for everyone, regardless of age, ability, or fitness level.

Conclusion

Don't be discouraged if you haven't seen the weight loss results you were hoping for yet. Weight loss is a complex process influenced by many factors beyond exercise alone. Celebrate the stronger, more flexible body you've cultivated through your practice. Notice how your energy levels have improved, your posture has changed, and you're more in tune with your body's needs. These are all significant victories on your path to better health.

Consistency is key. Stick with your chair yoga routine, gradually increasing the intensity and duration as you feel comfortable. Combine your practice with mindful eating habits, and be patient with yourself. Your body is undergoing positive changes, even if they're not immediately visible on the scale.

As we conclude this amazing journey together, thank you for your presence, dedication, and incredible resilience. Remember, yoga is a lifelong journey, not a destination. There will be ups and downs, triumphs and challenges—all part of the beautiful, messy human experience. Embrace it all with an open heart, knowing each step moves you forward.

If you've found value in this book, consider sharing your experience with others who might need that extra nudge to start their own chair yoga journey. Your words can inspire change and spread the joy of chair yoga to even more people.

Here's to your continued growth, wellness, and joy through chair yoga!

INDEX OF POSES

Index of Poses

REFERENCES

Bonura, K. B., & Tenenbaum, G. (2014). Effects of yoga on psychological health in older adults. *Journal of Physical Activity and Health*, *11*(7), 1334–1341. https://doi.org/10.1123/jpah.2012-0365

Chen, K.-M., Chen, M.-H., Hong, S.-M., Chao, H.-C., Lin, H.-S., & Li, C.-H. (2008). Physical fitness of older adults in senior activity centers after 24-week silver yoga exercises. *Journal of Clinical Nursing*, *17*(19), 2634–2646. https://doi.org/10.1111/j.1365-2702.2008.02338.x

Ekhat Yoga Team. (n.d.). *Hatha yoga*. Ekhart Yoga. https://www.ekhartyoga.com/resources/styles/hatha-yoga#:~:text=A%20yoga%20class%20described%20as

Gao, Y., Wang, J.-Y., Ke, F., Tao, R., Liu, C., & Yang, S.-Y. (2022). Effectiveness of Aromatherapy Yoga in Stress Reduction and Sleep Quality Improvement among Chinese Female College Students: A Quasi-Experimental Study. *Healthcare (Basel, Switzerland)*, *10*(9), 1686. https://doi.org/10.3390/healthcare10091686

Georg Feuerstein. (2013). *The yoga tradition: its history, literature, philosophy, and practice*. Hohm Press.

Hartfiel, Latha, Vedapriya, Tamilselvan, Mathangi D., & Balamadhuwanthi. (2012). Effect of chair yoga on heart rate variability, perceived stress, and sleep quality among nursing professionals from a tertiary care hospital. *Biomedicine*, *43*(01), 499–503. https://doi.org/10.51248/.v43i01.2292

Iyengar, B. K. S. (2014). *BKS iyengar yoga the path to holistic health*. Dorling Kindersley Ltd.

Kanaya, A. M., Araneta, M. R. G., Pawlowsky, S. B., Barrett-Connor, E., Grady, D., Vittinghoff, E., Schembri, M., Chang, A., Carrion-Petersen, M. L., Coggins, T., Tanori, D., Armas, J. M., & Cole, R. J. (2014). Restorative yoga and metabolic risk factors: The Practicing Restorative Yoga vs. Stretching for the Metabolic Syndrome (PRYSMS) randomized trial. *Journal of Diabetes and Its Complications*, *28*(3), 406–412. https://doi.org/10.1016/j.jdiacomp.2013.12.001

Kaoverii Weber, K. (2022, May 6). *Teaching yoga...despite the effects of gravity*. Subtle Yoga. https://subtleyoga.com/teaching-yoga-despite-gravity/

Klempel, N., Blackburn, N. E., McMullan, I. L., Wilson, J. J., Smith, L., Cunningham, C., O'Sullivan, R., Caserotti, P., & Tully, M. A. (2021). The effect of chair-based exercise on physical function in older adults: A systematic review and meta-analysis. *International Journal of Environmental Research and Public Health*, *18*(4), 1902. https://doi.org/10.3390/ijerph18041902

Lam, H. L., Li, W. T. V., Laher, I., & Wong, R. Y. (2020). Effects of Music Therapy on Patients with Dementia—A Systematic Review. *Geriatrics*, *5*(4), 62. https://doi.org/10.3390/geriatrics5040062

Lee, M., Lee, J., Park, B.-J., & Miyazaki, Y. (2015). Interaction with indoor plants may reduce psychological and physiological stress by suppressing autonomic nervous system activity in young adults: a randomized crossover study. *Journal of Physiological Anthropology*, *34*(1). https://doi.org/10.1186/s40101-015-0060-8

Noradechanunt, C., Worsley, A., & Groeller, H. (2017). Thai Yoga improves physical function and well-being in older adults: A randomized controlled trial. *Journal of Science and Medicine in Sport*, *20*(5), 494–501. https://doi.org/10.1016/j.jsams.2016.10.007

Nourish Yoga Training Content Team. (2021). *How to: Chair yoga – nourish yoga training*. Nourishyogatraining.com. https://nourishyogatraining.com/how-to-chair-yoga/#:~:text=It

Park, J., McCaffrey, R., Newman, D., Cheung, C., & Hagen, D. (2014). The effect of sit "N" fit chair yoga among community-dwelling older adults with osteoarthritis. *Holistic Nursing Practice*, *28*(4), 247–257. https://doi.org/10.1097/hnp.0000000000000034

Scaravelli, V. (2018). *Awakening the spine*. HarperCollins.

Singleton, M. (2010). *Yoga body: The origins of modern posture practice*. Oxford University Press.

Thomas, M. H., & Burns, S. P. (2016). Increasing Lean Mass and Strength: A Comparison of High Frequency Strength Training to Lower Frequency Strength Training. *International Journal of Exercise Science*, *9*(2), 159–167. https://www.ncbi.nlm.nih.gov/pmc/articles/PMC4836564/

Tran, M. D., Holly, R. G., Lashbrook, J., & Amsterdam, E. A. (2001). Effects of hatha yoga practice on the health-related aspects of physical fitness. *Preventive Cardiology*, *4*(4), 165–170. https://doi.org/10.1111/j.1520-037x.2001.00542.x

Zak Morris, S. (2020, August 30). *Essential program: Posture & flexibility*. Yoga Vista TV. https://yogavista.tv/articles/essential-program-posture-flexibility/

www.ingramcontent.com/pod-product-compliance
Lightning Source LLC
Chambersburg PA
CBHW080421030426
42335CB00020B/2541